THE DOCTOR

IN COLONIAL AMERICA

T̲H̲E̲ DOCTOR

IN COLONIAL AMERICA

ZACHARY B. FRIEDENBERG, M.D.

Rutledge Books, Inc.

Danbury, CT

Front cover artwork used with permission by Parke-Davis Company,
    Warner Lambert Subsidiary.

Back cover picture courtesy of College of Physicians, Philadelphia.

Rutledge Books, Inc.
107 Mill Plain Road, Danbury, CT 06811
1-800-278-8533

Manufactured in the United States of America

Cataloging in Publication Data
Friedenberg, Zachary B.
    The Doctor in Colonial America

    ISBN: 1-887750-93-2

    1. Physicians -- United States -- Biography.
2. Medicine -- History -- 18th Century

610.92   98-65792

Contents

PREFACE

In preparation for a difficult surgical operation, one is dependent on many skilled individuals to provide support, in addition to sophisticated equipment and imaging devices. At such times, an inquiring thought quickly crosses the mind: how was such a task approached when this skilled help and technological assistance were not available? The thought is quickly put out of mind by the pressures of the moment.

As an orthopaedic surgeon in a university hospital in Philadelphia, whose time has been spent in an active surgical practice, medical research, and teaching of medical students, orthopaedic residents and practicing physicians, I frequently—albeit briefly—pondered this question. In later years, a reduced workload provided me an opportunity to research and answer this recurrent question, of how the physicians and surgeons in Colonial America managed these problems in their era.

The story of our struggle for independence and the political philosophies of our early statesmen, which even now are models for statecraft throughout the world, captured my imagination even as a young high school student. I continue to savor this period and view these statesmen as model heroes. Initially this interest was fostered by a high school teacher in New York City, still well remembered, Miss Florence Myers. Her teaching of this period to an impressionable student made an indelible mark which persisted throughout my life and now is requited.

Military hospitals and medicine during the American Revolutionary War resonated throughout my experiences during the Second World War when I served two and a half years in a forward military hospital in Africa and Europe, so that war injuries, working under difficult circumstances, and the conduct of physicians in forward installations, as well as military hospital tactics, are well known to me.

I continue my work as a physician and teacher at this time.

Zachary B. Friedenberg, M.D.

ACKNOWLEDGMENTS

The College of Physicians in Philadelphia, founded in 1787, itself a part of the medical history of early America, was my primary resource. At my disposal was their collection of over one-half million books, letters and pamphlets on the history of medicine. To the College and their cooperative staff, I owe a deep debt of gratitude.

The Public Record Office in Kew, Surrey, in Britain and the Wellcome Library in London willingly provided me with assistance, as did the British Army Medical Historical Museum at Keogh Barracks near Aldershot.

Lastly, I am indebted to Kathie for important suggestions that improved the clarity and continuity of the text.

ABOUT THE AUTHOR

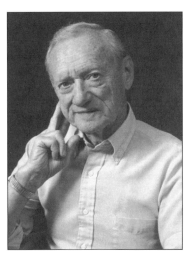

During Dr. Zachary Friedenberg's education, the war clouds thickened, and when he graduated medical school, Hitler's blitzkrieg had subdued the European Continent. He soon found himself in North Africa, Italy, France and Germany as an army surgeon in various forward surgical hospitals.

Once discharged, Dr. Friedenberg, as a well experienced military surgeon continued his interrupted formal education to become an orthopaedic surgeon in a major academic center.

Surgical research, teaching and surgical practice totally engulfed his professional life for many years. Yet in spite of diversions such as underwater photography, sailing and worldwide travel, something in his soul yearned to be expressed. Dr. Friedenberg had no choice but to retreat to centuries past, and repeat the slow and painful ascent of his medical predecessors up the ladder of time.

INTRODUCTION

This book is not intended just for a medically educated readership. At first, this was to be the focus, but medical practice in Colonial America was so intertwined with the political, religious, and cultural aspects of a new vibrant country rebelling against the mother country, that the tapestry would be threadbare if medicine were to be separated from the political unrest, the challenges of establishing a new political system, and the crude efforts of an inexperienced Continental Congress trying to establish a medical and hospital system for an army yet to be organized and which would be involved in battles from Quebec in the north to Georgia in the south. Add to this a burgeoning population, shifting westward, and the problems appear insurmountable.

This book, about the development of medicine in America, can best be understood from a historical, not a medical, perspective. The intricacies of medicine, medical vocabulary, and what little of technology that was present in the eighteenth century, tax the comprehension of the reader far less than understanding medical articles in the lay press at this time.

As much as possible, I have sought to depend on original articles published in the eighteenth century as reference material. It was my hope that this would permit a fresh approach to the subject, but, of course, it was not possible to exclude the many informative articles by others written more recently for which, I hope, I have given proper credit.

By immersing myself in the original medical literature with a sympathetic understanding of a doctor's problems, I have experienced his frustrations as he grappled for a diagnosis and treatment of his sick patient with the limited knowledge available to him.

Many of the books and pamphlets reviewed were originally published in Britain and within the year brought to America and reprinted, finding their way to the bookshelves of America. They were read by other people than doctors. Thomas Jefferson believed that every citizen should understand anatomy as part of a general education in natural philosophy.

Beginning in the early years of the eighteenth century and until the advent of the war, many American students were educated in Edinburgh and elsewhere in Britain, and, once established in practice, they continued to correspond with their teachers, fellow students and friends in Britain. Their transatlantic letters discussed new medical ideas and sought help for perplexing cases, so that a well-traveled bridge of information exchange continued even throughout the war, when they learned that many of their teachers and fellow students were sympathetic to the American cause.

Their understanding of disease and practice of medicine was founded on British medical books because of a common language, medical training and kinship. For an understanding of American medicine, it was necessary to consult many references from Britain and to understand medicine as it was practiced there, modified somewhat by the wide expanse of the land, the absence of a class system, and the inferior training of some American doctors.

The times were turbulent. America was rebelling against the strongest military power in the world, a country that had sent expeditionary forces throughout Europe, to the West Indies, and had recently successfully triumphed over the French in North America. Its army medical department was lead by top quality physicians with long experience in military medicine. In contrast, the American medical scene can best be described in the words of James Tilton, M.D., an American army physician who served throughout the war: "It would be shocking to humanity to relate the history of our general hospitals in the years 1777-8 when it swallowed up at least one half of our army, owing to a fatal tendency in the system...."

Today, the practice of medicine is increasingly based on scientific discipline. The fanciful theories, therapeutic logic and rationalizations are gone. For those who have a nostalgic yearning for the simplicity of life and the family togetherness of that century—beware! Readers will learn that health, well-being, freedom from pain and suffering were not included in the blessings of this society. Instead, the reader will discover that rampant disease, disabling injuries and sudden death were the realities to be faced. Successful treatment of disease and longevity were not included in the contract between the physician and the patient.

CHAPTER ONE

MEDICAL PRACTICE

"A review of the mode of living of our forefathers, if it is to be useful should be sympathetic in its attitude. The lapse of time often obscures the difficulties surrounding a former generation and we are apt to smile at curities where a just estimate should rather leave us to marvel that so much was accomplished with so little." [1]

For those who follow the progress of medicine and its recent dependence on biochemistry, molecular biology and electronic imaging techniques, medical practice in the past without such assistance seems impossible. How did the physician arrive at a diagnosis without these tools, indeed without a stethoscope or a means to measure blood pressure? Treatment presented even a greater problem, and there were few effective therapies.

The thought presents itself that perhaps treatment by the doctor contributed nothing to the cure of the patient. Like the primitive medicine man, the physician was someone who appeared on the scene to accept responsibility from the family and, shouldering it himself, guided the patient through difficult circumstances, relieving the anxieties of the relatives and family. Rarely did he further the healing process which was destined to go one way or another depending on the virulence of the disease and the resistance of the patient.

Before the eighteenth century and continuing into the following century, doctors were not expected to combat the ravages of epidemics. This was a score to be settled between a sinful community and the Almighty, and if an individual survived, it was not due to a skillful physician but to the mercy of God. Daniel Defoe wrote in 1665:

> "Amongst the many calamities with which the Almighty is pleased to visit the children of men in order to reduce them to a just sense of their own weakness and entire dependence upon Him...are those contagious distempers which an offended God sometimes suffers to rage among the people."[2]

In truth, such plague victims should not be treated to thwart God's will. In *The Dreadful Visitation of the Plague in London in 1665*, Defoe states the usual numbers of deaths in London were 240-300 per week. As the death rate rose, the nobility and gentry fled the city and throughout the summer the death rate remained at greater than 1,000 per week.

An interesting sidelight to this epidemic was its effect on the nature of London's inhabitants. Style-conscious peacocks affected a simple dress, people became very civil to each other, class lines blurred, works of charity increased, crime in the streets was no longer evident and the churches were overcrowded.

In America, too, in this period, the physician was called only after peace with the Lord was established. People sought the Lord for their health as well as their political and moral problems. In a textbook of medicine which was handwritten in Pennsylvania about 1770, the first statement under the heading of preserving one's health is, "...fear God and follow a calm, moderate life, and with the blessing of providence you will preserve your health."[3]

When an eight-year-old boy by the name of Bumstead fell from a gallery in the meetinghouse and broke his arm and shoulder in the Massachusetts Bay Colony, treatment was committed to the Lord by prayer with a desire that the place where His people assembled to worship Him might not be defiled with blood. It pleased the Lord, so this child was soon perfectly recovered.[4]

People saw God's hand in each passing event. The smallpox epidemic and other diseases introduced by the Massachusetts Colony, which decimated the Indian population, were sent by the Lord to tame the savage heart and teach them the need to fear God, chasten them for their sins—and make room for the pilgrims.[5] When disease struck the settlers, it was punishment for their misdeeds and the wicked took the righteous with them. If the physician succeeded in healing the patient, it was because of God's intercession. When a physician is needed to be selected, the physician must be God-fearing.[6]

It was observed that a shipload of new settlers would precipitate a disease epidemic. In Salem in 1629, "...an infection that grue among the passengers at sea, spread also among them a shore..." and the General Court of the Massachusetts Bay Colony, in December 1629, set a limit on the number of passengers in each ship "...in proportion to its burthen..." to avoid overcrowding.[7]

Michael Wigglesworth, a physician and clergyman, wrote in 1662:

Our healthfull dayes are at an end,
and sicknesses come on
From yeer to yeer becaus our hearts
Away from God are gone.
New England where for many yeers

To Preserve Health: A handwritten medicine textbook which instructs one to "...fear God and follow a calm, moderate life..."

you scarcely heard a cough,
and where physicians had no work
Now finds them work enough[8]

Some of this community guilt was still evident in the latter eigh-teenth century in Philadelphia during the yellow fever epidemic in 1793, where 50-100 persons died of the disease daily. The threat of sudden death to each individual altered the behavior of people toward their neighbors and to the community.[9]

Before this, in the early part of the eighteenth century, Cotton Mather, the liberal, outspoken clergyman in Boston and the physician Zabdiel Boylston teamed together to pressure the community to accept inoculation as a preventive of smallpox. A mighty tide of resistance to this treatment swelled, supported by churchmen, political officeholders and the press, as well as doctors decrying the new treatment. Saving people from death was interfering with the will of God who had cast down such a plague to smite the people of New England for their irrev-erence. Moreover, the treatment itself by transferring pox from a dis-eased individual to a healthy neighbor was diabolical interference. Boylston was assaulted in the street, his house attacked by a mob and a bomb was thrown into his parlor where his wife was sitting.

* * * * * *

In Europe, physicians and surgeons maintained a separate identi-ty. The physician traced his roots to Galen and was a highly respected individual often working in a university setting and distinguished by his academic garments and later by the gold-headed cane. The sur-geon filled a void, caring for patients outside the physician's sphere. There were wounds to be healed, amputations that must be done, bleeding to be staunched, bones to be set and teeth to be pulled. A class of untrained individuals cared for such problems. Known as barber surgeons, bonesetters or simply surgeons, their knowledge was empirical and passed down from father to son.

> "I am called on many a behalf
> Can make a curative salve,—
> Can heal fresh wounds with right good grace,
> And old wounds, too, as well as bone breaks;
> Heal the French pox and needle a cataract,
> Quench Anthony's Fire and teeth extract;
> Likewise shave, massage, and trim,
> And open veins at anybody's whim."[10]

Surgeons gained an elevated status through the work of Ambroise Paré who studied wounds in France during the Thirty Years' War in the seventeenth century. Paré himself was originally an apprentice to a barber surgeon. Charles Wiseman, at that time in England, also gained eminence in treating wounds and kept a journal of the results of his treatment. It remained, however, for John Hunter and his surgical research experiments to lift surgery from a mechanical craft to the status of a profession, soon to be organized in London as the Royal College of Surgeons.

Thomas Buckle, in his History of Civilization, wrote, "I have only one more name to add to this splendid catalogue of the great Scotsmen of the eighteenth century. But it is the name of a man who for comprehensive and original genius comes immediately after Adam Smith, and must be placed far above any philosopher whom Scotland has produced. I mean, of course, John Hunter, whose only fault was an occasional obscurity, not merely of language, but of thought." To Sir James Mackenzie, "Hunter is the Shakespeare of Medicine. To the many American students who studied with him, lived in his home, assisted with his experiments, Hunter was equated with Harvey, Bacon and Newton."[11]

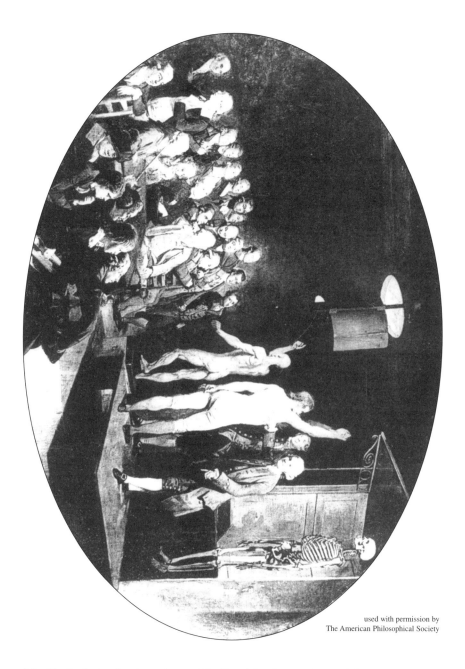

used with permission by
The American Philosophical Society

John Hunter instructing in anatomy at the Royal Academy using models.

In America, the separation of physicians and surgeons never developed. John Morgan, the first professor of physic at the College of Philadelphia, which became the University of Pennsylvania after the War for Independence, suggested in an address at the time the school opened in May, 1765, that the practice of medicine should be divided into physicians, surgeons, and apothecaries. John Jones, professor of surgery at Kings' College (later the College of Physicians, Columbia University), in New York City disagreed and spoke against this concept, indicating a doctor should take care of all patients regardless of complaints.[12]

The American physician practiced both medicine and surgery during this period and for the next 150 years. This practice was not ordained by any individual or organization, but was a natural consequence of the American scene. There were few cities; the first United States census in 1790 showed Philadelphia with 45,000 inhabitants, New York with 33,000, and Boston with 18,000; most people lived in remote farms, and the frontier stretched farther westward each year. A handful of doctors educated in medical schools, many who trained as apprentices, and assorted other "healers" supported the widely separated communities and were required to provide all the services. In the classless American social structure, the sharp distinction between physician and surgeon present in Europe was blurred and lost.

* * * * * *

In the absence of scientific knowledge about disease causation, the physicians embraced a holistic theory of disease to explain all maladies. The precedent for a theory embracing all illnesses goes back to Galen, whose theories influenced medical thought and treatment for centuries. Galen taught that disease occurs when there is an imbalance of the four body fluids: blood, phlegm, yellow bile and black bile. The English physician Thomas Sydenham modified this theory by describing an external morbidity which upset the balance when it entered the body and the resulting symptoms were the efforts of the patient to throw off the disease.[13] When possible, Sydenham taught specificity in making a diagnosis.

Medical leaders attracted disciples to their theories and confrontation between the followers of one theory and another pervaded medical literature. Herman Boerhaave, the famous Dutch physician and teacher of the eighteenth century, like Galen, attributed all diseases to an alteration of body fluids. He recognized that a morbid exterior element entered the body to contaminate the fluids and cause symptoms—vomiting, sweating and diarrhea—which were efforts of the sick to discharge the unwanted element. Treatment according to this theory should assist the body in ridding itself of the toxic substance and this was accomplished by bleeding, purgatives, and medications to cause discharge of fluids. To allow the toxic substance to be expelled from the pores of the skin, the patient must be confined to bed with fresh cool air to be excluded by closed windows and doors and drawn curtains so that a sweat occurred. In a routine physical examination, the physician relied most on the pulse, noting its rate, hardness, softness, the thickness of the vessel wall and its pulsatile quality. Any coating of the tongue was ascribed significance. The skin color and eyes were noted for jaundice. The urine quantity, color, odor, and viscosity was noted. A thermometer was rarely used.

The pulse was thought to transmit a wealth of information. Fast pulses are to be treated by a regimen of cold applications; slow pulses, by heat. A hard pulse is the result of obstruction of the vessel, and the proper pulse rate is determined, among other variables, by the latitude. The pulse rate was thought to be highest at the equator, lowest at $90°$ of latitude; in England it is at 70 beats. To more accurately study the pulse, a pulse watch was described which ran for 60 seconds. The Chinese method of examining the pulse was thought superior to the Western method of pulse examination. The pulse must be felt in the morning, when the patient is fasting, by a physician who is healthful and free of cares. The left hand of the patient is placed on a pillow while the second and third fingers of the examiner studied the pulse.[14] In America and Britain, many diagnoses were made by feeling the pulse, but it is doubtful if the Chinese method prevailed in the pragmatic Western culture.

The urine sample could be further tested by adding acids or alkalis. If bloodletting was part of the treatment, the character of the drawn blood in the basin would be noted. Was it thin, viscous, light, dark or frothy? The only laboratory instruments were the watch and sometimes a thermometer. Balance of body fluids could be restored by getting rid of the toxic fluids and then providing the addition of medicines.

By the end of the century much less emphasis was placed on the balance of body humors and more on the toxic substances surrounding people. The air could be contaminated and the words "infected" and "contagious" were in wide use.

The explosive outbreak of an epidemic and the passage of disease within families and to their neighbors was usually described as a result of impure or toxic air, but to some it meant passage of a more specific substance which was called "contagium vivum". For example, a tiny but visible mite associated with scabies was known as the cause of the disease. Here was a specific agent causing a specific disease. It was possible that the invisible animaliculae seen floating under Van Leeuwenhoek's microscope might spread disease as well as the itch mite.[15]

In 1774, William Buchan in England wrote a popular book on health, "addressed to the populace", on how to live the healthy life. Unwholesome air was identified as the most common cause of disease. People were not aware of its noxious quality and how it deteriorated when too cold or hot or when too moist. Air was deemed bad in hospitals, jails, and in the holds of ships, and people contracted disease when crowded together. Sick people should be avoided, viewing the corpse was dangerous and graveyards should be given a wide berth. People should dress in loose clothing so the pores would not be clogged. Exercise, cold baths and cleanliness were recommended and "...no person who labours under an incurable malady ought to marry."

We are shocked to learn that one half of the children born in Great Britain at this time died before the age of twelve. This is far higher than the death rate in animals in this period and Buchan accused parents of mistreating children. "How can a mother be so ignorant to not know the proper care of her child? This is not true in the animal kingdom. The mother that brings up her child by proxy,...abandons the child and hardly deserves the name of a parent." They should not send their children off to school at too young an age and should give them more attention than they pay to their kennels and stables. The author obviously had a practice of wealthy families, but his ideas of health are advanced and refreshing even though based on the wrong premise.[16]

The concept of a unified theory of disease espoused by Galen, whether due to imbalance of the humors or the theories of toxic air, received an impetus beginning in the seventeenth century after the rapid advances that were made in the physical sciences. Newton's all-embracing theory of gravity was so widely applied to explain so many physical phenomena, that a parallel in medicine was sought, a theory that would explain all disease and lead to a common drug for treatment. What those in medicine failed to appreciate was the derivation of Newton's theory from scientific experiments, supported by mathematical equations, not armchair theorizing.

Most prominent physicians elaborated their own theories of disease. William Cullen, of the Edinburgh Infirmary, developed a theory of disease which was widely accepted in America, having been brought back by the many American students attending the school at Edinburgh. Cullen called his theory "solidism", as it no longer ascribed the diseased state to a fluid contamination or imbalance, but due to an affection of the nerves.[17]

In America, Benjamin Rush taught that there was only one disease that nature inflicted on mankind. It was expressed in different forms and might seem to be several diseases. The disease occurred as a result of "morbid excitement", which caused over- excitement of the blood vessels. Presumably, excitement implied increased vascular flow and proliferation and engorgement of the vessels resulting in increased heat of a part and fever within the patient. Treatment of disease, therefore, demanded a low diet, purges, bleeding, and keeping the patient relaxed.[18] Regardless of theory, the treatment prescribed always depended on the same repetition of bleeding, purges, and the same medications.

One of Rush's apprentices, upon entering practice, extended Rush's general theory of disease, with a cure for cancer which he widely advertised, using present day marketing techniques. When he asked George Washington for a testimonial, Washington replied that if such an important drug worked, it should not be a secret, and further advised that testimonials ought to come from cured patients, rather than national personages.[19]

In America, Rush was the extreme proponent of rationalism in medicine. All the ills of mankind must fit into a single theory. He taught that there was only one disease in the world and he made the point so forcibly in his lectures that his students feared to question his authority.[20] This was dogmatism in medicine just as it was in theology, pure speculation with no factual basis, and it was an impenetrable barrier to medical progress.

Thomas Jefferson had a keen interest in medicine. He believed that every individual should have a basic understanding of how his body functions and, as a youth, he studied the anatomy text of Cheselden. To Thomas Randolph, his future son-in-law, studying law and politics in Britain, he recommended he travel to the University of

Edinburgh to study anatomy. At the same time, Jefferson scoffed at the theories of disease espoused by the leading doctors in Europe and America. When his grandson was to travel to Philadelphia to study medicine, Jefferson encouraged him to devote his time to anatomy and botany, the basic sciences, but to avoid theory.[21]

Jefferson offered advice to medical students: "His mind must be strong indeed, if, rising above juvenile credulity, it can maintain a wise infidelity against the authority of his instructors and the bewitching delusions of their theories."[22]

The physical sciences had already accepted the experimental approach, but medicine lagged behind. Morgagni in Padua in 1761 was studying the results of a large number of autopsies and relating his findings to the symptoms of the patient before death, so defining specific disease entities. Here was the first glimmer of cause and effect, separated from theory.

In America, Thomas Bond at Pennsylvania Hospital was familiar with the work of Morgagni and emphasized autopsies, but the influence of Rush, his many writings and his political and personal reputation were so great that medicine in America was stagnant, dominated by his ideas until beyond 1820.

Some important medical information had been published and was slowly becoming known and accepted throughout Europe and America. Harvey had demonstrated the course of the circulation of the blood; Vesalius emphasized the importance of anatomical dissection; and Paré had written his volumes on wound care. From this foundation of knowledge, important advances were in the offing. John Hunter and Sir John Pringle lead the way in eighteenth-century research, and Cullen and Monro in Edinburgh began to teach medicine by bedside teaching rather than from textbooks. However, it was not until the following century that medical advances flowered with such giants as Pasteur, Virchow and Lister.

In all of the major European cities, hospitals were established bringing together physcians who compared their theories and results. It was after this that physicians and surgeons were organized into societies and medical journals were published. At the onset of this period in America, there were few journals and no societies. The first hospital, Pennsylvania Hospital, was established in 1752 in Philadelphia. The medical traditions in Europe were transplanted to this country with the medical students returning from their schools and hospitals overseas. Slowly the accumulating information from Europe came to the larger cities and penetrated into the wilderness of America, where it had to weather the prewar political turmoil and came to a halt with the onset of hostilities. The importation of medical ideas and students to America was amply repaid by the new freedoms and democratic theories later exported to Europe to question their political structures.

The experienced physician, not tied to dogma, could sort out certain diseases which presented themselves with a chain of symptoms and followed a specific course. In such cases, his treatment and understanding were divorced from any theory. Diseases presented differently in different seasons, in different countries, in isolated individuals or in crowded cities or military camps, in different age groups and often with specific symptoms which allowed them to be characterized. Manifest symptoms such as the rash of measles, the skin encrustations of smallpox, the membrane coating the throat in diphtheria, or the jaundice of yellow fever signaled a specific entity, the course of which could be anticipated. Although the experienced, observant and perceptive physician might adhere to a theory, he also separated out such diseases for specific treatment unrelated to any theory.

The physician thus employed a two-tiered system for making a diagnosis. The experienced physician recognized a train of events and related it to an entity whose course and treatment he was familiar with even though its pathology and etiology were beyond his knowledge.

If he didn't recognize the condition, he would fall back on a theory. In either event, the treatment was likely to be the same.

* * * * * * *

Physicians of the eighteenth century were intellectual leaders and formed the largest single group in the Royal Society. Boerhaave, Haller, Linnaeus, Hunter, Lind and others were educated in botany, comparative anatomy, chemistry, mathematics, astronomy and physics. It is therefore not unexpected that this enlightened group sought other ways of explaining disease outside of the constrained parameters of a theory.

Medical conditions seen by the physician at that time included diagnoses of hospital, camp or jail fever, putrid fever, bilious fever, yellow fever, dysentery or the bloody flux, pleuritic fever, consumption, scrofula, syphilis and venereal diseases, or arthritis.

Hospital, camp or jail fever was thought to result from putrid air when people were packed into a confined space. In addition to its spread in crowded hospitals, it was also observed on transport ships and was recognized as a contagion, spread from one individual to another. Fever, nausea, headache and backache, occasionally diarrhea, and petechiae—or blotched skin—were present. Death or recovery occurred in fourteen to twenty days. Autopsy showed glandular suppuration, sometimes a brain abscess or mortification of the intestines.[23] This was obviously an infection, most likely typhus, perhaps typhoid fever, septicemia or a blood stream infection, perhaps in a patient with a vitamin C deficiency. Sending a patient to a hospital for any reason could result in such an infection and was often a death sentence.

Sir John Pringle published evidence and concluded that hospital, jail or camp fever were the same disease. Some English soldiers in Flanders deserted to the French and, having later fought with the

Jacobites and Scots at the battle of Culloden, were captured by the British as deserters and imprisoned; they soon developed jail fever. Camp and hospital fever raged after this battle, and Pringle showed that all three diseases presented common symptoms and followed the same course. Moreover, he published regulations which, when enforced, could control the spread of these diseases. Upon discharge no prisoner must carry out or wear the clothes he had worn, but the old clothes were to be burned; clothes of those executed in prison must not be given away, but also burned; and, finally, before a prisoner was brought to court, they should be cleansed and put on new clothes. Judges on the bench, hearing the cases of diseased prisoners, died of jail fever contracted from the prisoners before the bar. There were no regulations attempting to control the spread among inmates in the prison. Pringle also described cross infection in hospitals and was one of the first to use the term antiseptic, which he described as acids or distilled spirits or alcohol.

Such an inquiring and perceptive mind must have considered a living agent as the source of spreading of disease, particularly as others had conjectured a contagium vivum or animaliculae as the agent of disease. However, the leap of the mind to form a new idea fell short and Pringle still believed in foul air as the basis for disease and rejected live organisms as a cause.[24] During the American Revolutionary War, Pringle's ideas were known in America, but enforcement by military officers was slack or nonexistent.

The bloody flux was one of several forms of dysentery. Fever was present and the skin was dry and dehydrated. This could include any intestinal infection, even typhoid. Military campsites were often the areas of such a contagion. Good sanitation in a military camp was known to limit the number of patients and arrest epidemics. The term "infectious" was first used by Pringle in referring to this disease.

Pringle, in his earlier years, was chief physician of the British army in the campaigns in the Netherlands and northern France, and made the observation that troops on the move were healthier than those in encampments, as fresh privies were dug at each bivouac and fresh hay was collected for bedding material. Moreover, the adjacent streams weren't corrupted when the encampment was brief and filth didn't collect in the campground. He also noted that soldiers fared badly in hospitals compared to those who remained in camp. He ordered company officers to dig deeper privies, particularly in summer, and to layer them with soil daily.[25] This message was only belatedly learned by American physicians and military staff officers, after the loss of thousands of lives in the American military forces.

Bilious fever was a remitting type of fever with its highest incidence in the fall and often was fatal. Symptoms were chills, fever, headaches, loose stools, bilious vomiting, hemorrhage and nose bleeds with some patients showing jaundice. This might be one of several diseases, including hepatitis or yellow fever. This condition was to be separated from autumnal or tertian fever which could be malaria.

Smallpox was easily identified by skin crusts and its epidemic nature. For centuries it had decimated populations. It was recognized that having survived one attack of smallpox, an individual would be immune to this disease for the remainder of his life. A person with a pock-marked face was fortunate as he was immune from smallpox.

In 1677 the first printed medical article in America was written by Thomas Thacher, Minister of the Old South Church in Boston, and was directed to the public giving advice on the treatment of smallpox and measles. His recommendations were of a general nature.

Smallpox inoculation (not vaccination) was practiced from time immemorial in Ciraffia, Georgia, and the countries bordering the Caspian Sea. The practice had spread to Constantinople in the fifteenth century, was neglected and then disappeared. It was revived again at the end of the seventeenth century and its practice spread throughout Turkey and Greece. Independently it was discovered in

Bengal, China, and on the coast and in the interior of Africa, from whence the practice spread to Algiers, Tunis and Tripoli.

In these areas, the practice was to place a crust from the skin of a patient recovering from the disease on the arm or leg of the person to be inoculated and scarify the area with a knife. In China, it was not inoculated, but the crust was placed on a piece of cotton which was packed into a nostril where the virus was inspired.

In 1713, Emanuel Timone, a Greek doctor, described the procedure to an English physician, Dr. Woodward, but no action was taken. Timone wrote that he had been inoculating for eight years and observed only two deaths as a result of the inoculations.

This information was reported in Western Europe on several other occasions, but again the idea did not spread. James Pilarni, another Greek physician who had disapproved of the practice was later convinced and wrote an apology in Latin, which was printed in Venice in 1715. A Thessalian woman, practicing in Constantinople, claimed to have inoculated 6000 people in 1713, many of them English, French or Dutch merchants.

It was left for Lady Worley Montague, the wife of the English ambassador to the Ottoman Empire, to promote the practice in Western Europe on her return to England. In Turkey, she had her only son of five years inoculated, and on her return to England she inoculated her daughter. Her example soon spread to her friends and others. The College of Physicians in London experimented on six convicts about to be hanged, who were spared so that their post-inoculation course could be followed.

The Princess of Wales became a convert and had two of her daughters inoculated; she in turn convinced the Queen of Denmark and the Princess of Hesse-Cassel to be inoculated in 1722. The initiative seemed to be taken by women arranging for the inoculation of their children.

Physicians were pitted against each other; some supporting the idea, some proscribing it. Again we note that the reason for denying the inoculation was because it was contrary to the wishes of God to prevent an Almighty-sent epidemic. Inoculation would bring down the wrath of God. The secretary of the Royal Society kept records of those who contracted the disease after inoculation. He noted that only one in ninety-five died of the inoculation, whereas one in five-to-seven infected persons died of a smallpox infection. Thus, the relative safety of the procedure was established, but evidence for inoculation to prevent the disease was still lacking.[26]

The practice of inoculation spread to America with incredible speed. Lady Montague returned to England in 1721 and inoculations in America began in the same year. It might be anticipated that such interference with nature would not flourish in New England with its rigid puritanical background and hostile opposition did quickly arise.

When news of the inoculation procedure in England reached Cotton Mather, a liberal clergyman, he became active in promoting it in Boston. In 1721 and 1722 Mather wrote articles on the procedure. He claimed to have known something about inoculation previously from questioning a black slave. In a letter to John Woodward of the British Museum in 1716, Mather writes, "...inquiring of my Negro man, Onesimus, who is a pretty intelligent fellow, whether he had the Small Pox; he answered both Yes and No: and then told me that he had undergone an operation which had given him something of the Small Pox and would forever preserve him from it; adding that it was often used among the Guramantese."[27]

Mather sought help from the physicians of Boston, but could find only one ally, Zabdiel Boylston. Mather of the clergy and Boylston, the physician, urged inoculation and started an inoculation drive in Boston. Many elderly people were inoculated in this group and five died, a somewhat greater mortality than reported by the Royal College.

The magistrates, reacting to vitriolic opposition from pamphlets and the newspapers, as well as the pulpit, forbade any further inoculations. In an article published in Boston, an anonymous author savagely attacked Mather.[28]

The author passionately abused Mather: "The Church ought to deliver him over to Satan for he deserves the highest censure, deserves to be scourged out of the country. The government ought to banish him. He should be pilloried and afterward stoned by the people." This attack probably arose from the pen of William Douglass, a Scottish physician who had emigrated to Boston and was a leader of the medical community. The ban against inoculation finally was lifted, although the clamor against it grew.

Boylston first inoculated his son and servants and on becoming more convinced and confident of the efficacy of the method inoculated 247 people in 1722. Other physicians inoculated thirty-nine others for a pool of 286 persons. During this period an epidemic of smallpox raged and 5,759 cases of smallpox were recorded in Boston of whom 804 died (about 15%), but in the 286 exposed inoculated group, only six died (2%).[29,30] Boylston's figures were confirmed in Charleston, South Carolina, which experienced a severe smallpox epidemic in 1730 traced to a British ship, London Frigate, which had brought infected slaves from Guinea. Of a pool of 623 inoculated people in Charleston, 16 died (3.6%); of 1675 smallpox victims not inoculated, 295 died (17.6%).[31]

In England, the Royal Society had established the relative safety of the inoculation, but did it prevent death when an inoculated individual was subjected to the disease? It thus remained for Boylston to show that those who were inoculated were protected against smallpox.[32]

In spite of his success, Boylston was called before the court. Later, he traveled to England where he was received as a hero and made a member of the Royal Society.

Washington had noted the military disasters of his armies due to smallpox and strongly advocated inoculation, and by the end of the war, the entire army was inoculated. In Virginia smallpox inoculation was made illegal. In a letter to Patrick Henry in Virginia, Washington wrote, "You will pardon my observation on the smallpox, because I know it is more destructive to an army in the natural way than the swords...." Later, in 1777, Washington wrote to John Augustus Washington in Virginia: "I congratulate you very sincerely on the happy passage of my sister and the rest of your family through the smallpox inoculation. Surely the daily instances which present themselves of the amazing benefits of inoculation must make converts of the most rigid opposers and bring repeal of the most impolitic law which restrains it."[33]

The approved method of inoculation in America suggested that the pustules be recovered from patients with a mild form of the disease. The recipient should be prepared for several days with a mild diet and one or two gentle purges, sometimes bathing beforehand. An incision just through the skin less than an inch in length was made in both arms in an area of the deltoid muscle of the shoulder. A thread impregnated with the crusts was inserted into the incision and the wound dressed daily. On the sixth or seventh day, when fever developed, the patient was put to bed. Wounds usually closed by the twentieth day, after formation of the pustule. Many variations of this method existed.[34]

Inoculation was the first step in a process which virtually eliminated smallpox worldwide. The era of inoculation was brief, but it prepared the public for the more recently developed vaccination of Jenner, who used cowpox rather than smallpox crusts to prevent smallpox. Edward Jenner, in rural Gloucestershire, England, like most physicians at this time was inoculating his patients with smallpox matter to prevent this disease, and was disturbed by the large number of his patients who failed to get a *take*, or local reaction, at the site of inoculation. When he studied his rate of successful inoculations with those of his colleagues in London or elsewhere, it compared very poorly.

Jenner had overheard dairymaids gossiping, stating they could not get smallpox because they once had cowpox. It was known to them from time immemorial and a vague opinion prevailed, "that dairy maids once having suffered an attack of cowpox were immune to smallpox." So widespread was this opinion in this dairy county that people who had suffered cowpox were sought out to nurse small-pox victims, with the knowledge they would not contract the disease.

Moreover, on further investigation, he found that some milkers in his community had suffered an attack of cowpox twenty-five or more years ago and had remained unscathed in spite of being exposed to numerous smallpox epidemics. Wherever cowpox appeared in a herd, farm owners assigned milkers who had recovered from smallpox or cowpox to milk the infected cows so that the business of the farm could proceed without interruption.[35]

Jenner began his studies of cowpox in 1775. This disease affects the udders and teats of cows causing swelling and pustules, and is easily transmitted to the dairymaids milking such cows. The infected milker developed itchy swelling of the fingers and hands which later formed pustules. About the ninth day after infection a low-grade fever and malaise occurred, after which there was a full recovery and the pustules did not cause permanent scars.

Jenner believed that the disease originated in horses who have a condition known to farriers as "The Grease", and is a festering of the heel of a horse. On this point Jenner was wrong and such transmis-sion was never proved.

He must now prove his suspicions. In 1796, "The first experiment was made upon a lad by the name of Phipps in whose arm a little Vaccine Virus* was inserted taken from the hand of a young woman who had been accidentally infected by a cow.

Notwithstanding the resemblance which the pustule thus excited on the boy's arm bore to variolous inoculation (smallpox), yet as the

---

* Jenner was using the term Virus as an infecting agent, not the present understanding of a virus as we know it.

22

indisposition attending it was barely perceptible, I could scarcely persuade myself the patient was secure from the Smallpox. However, on being inoculated some months afterward, it proved he was secure."[36]

In another inquiry Jenner states, "The more accurately to observe the progress of the infection, I selected a healthy boy eight years old for the purpose of INOCULATION FOR THE COWPOX. The matter was taken from a sore on the hand of a dairy maid who was infected from her master's cows, and it was inserted on the 14 of May 1796 into the arm of the boy by means of two superficial incisions, barely penetrating the cutis, each about half an inch long.

"On the seventh day he complained of uneasiness in the axilla and on the ninth he became a little chilly, lost his appetite, and had a slight head ache. During the whole of the day he was perceptibly indisposed and spent the night with some degree of restlessness, but on the following day, he was perfectly well.

"The appearance of the incisions in their progress to a state of maturation were much the same as when produced by variolous matter....

"In order to ascertain whether the boy after feeling so slight an affection of the system from the cowpox virus was secure from the contagion of the Small Pox, he was inoculated the first of July following, with variolous matter immediately taken from a pustule. Several slight punctures and incisions were made on both his arms and the matter was carefully inserted, but no disease followed." Jenner inoculated many people in his district—most between four and twelve years of age—to prove his theory, but used anecdotal rather than statistical evidence.[37,38]

Dr. Benjamin Waterhouse in Cambridge, Massachusetts, had followed Jenner's ideas and requested some cowpox material to be sent him in America. Dr. John Lettsom of the smallpox Inoculation Hospital in London, after conferring with Jenner, agreed to send the material. The first problem to be overcome was how the vaccine was to be transported in a three or more weeks' voyage across the Atlantic.

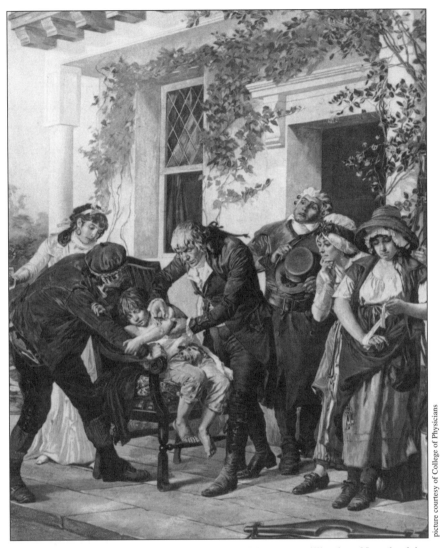

picture courtesy of College of Physicians

Painting of Jenner applying cowpox pustular material to an unwilling boy. Note the dairy maid bandaging her hand from which the material was taken.

Jenner suggested that the fluid be placed on a glass square and covered with a second piece of glass after which the edges would be sealed with sealing wax. Another suggestion was to infect two or three members of the crew or passengers with the vaccine and on the ninth day, when the pustule formed, inoculate the fluid into the arms of a second and third relay and thus arrive with it in America. In support of this latter method Lettsom stated he had heard of over 1700 people who were vaccinated by passing the infected cowpox material from person to person. Fortunately, the vaccine seemed to retain its potency even when dried. Doctors in England frequently moistened a piece of cotton dipped in the vaccine and allowed it to slowly dry in the air, not near a fire, and then rolled it up as a scroll and placed it in an envelope, to be used at a distant site.

It finally was sent across the Atlantic between glass squares in which form it was received by Waterhouse in 1799, only three years after Jenner's original experiments.

Cowpox was unknown in America and Waterhouse wrestled with his conscience about introducing a new distemper this side of the Atlantic. He had to be sure of the results of vaccination, and more than that, that no future unknown effects would develop. Waterhouse started at the beginning, repeating Jenner's experiments, and vaccinated the eight members of his family. Several months later he asked another physician to infect three of his vaccinated children with smallpox. They did not contract the disease and he proceeded to vaccinate several hundred people.

Contrary to the stormy reception given the smallpox inoculation in America over sixty years ago, its introduction created little furor. Benjamin Rush, the leading American physician, pronounced vaccination as the most useful discovery of the eighteenth century. John Adams wrote a letter to Waterhouse:

> From the President of the United States to
> Dr. Waterhouse, Quincy, Sept 10, 1800.
>
> Dear Sir,
>
> I have received and will communicate to the American

Academy of Arts and Sciences your *Prospects of Exterminating Small-Pox.*

I have read your history of the Kine-pock with great pleasure. Your zeal and industry in giving these experiments fair play in America deserve the thanks of all the friends of science and humanity.

To disarm the Small-Pox of it's contagion is an enterprise truly worthy of an HERCULES in medicine.

With great regard I am

Dear Sir, Your obliged friend,

and humble servant,

John Adams[39]

Later Waterhouse received a letter from President Jefferson:

From the President of the United States
Washington, Dec 25, 1800.

Dear Dr. Waterhouse,

Every friend of humanity must look with pleasure on this discovery by which one evil more is withdrawn from the condition of man....; and I pray you to accept my portion of the tribute due to you, and assurances of high consideration and respect, with which I am, Sir

Your most obedient humble servant

Thomas Jefferson[40]

Of course, there were critics who decried introducing "a bestial humor into the human frame" which undoubtedly would cause future untold problems. Waterhouse replied, "What may be the consequences after a long lapse of years of introducing into the human frame, cow's milk, beef steaks or a mutton chop?"[41]

In London 60,000 people were now vaccinated and four deaths were recorded, which probably were not related to cowpox, but perhaps the fluid was contaminated with virulent bacteria. Physicians in England celebrated with enthusiasm and ardor, the greatest "victory of medicine in recorded history—a discovery that surpasses the discovery of gunpowder, printing, the mariners compass and even the circulation of the blood."[42]

"Trophies and Statues have been erected to commemorate sanguinary deeds. Saul may have boasted of his thousands slain, and David of his ten thousands: But the altar of Jenner is not consecrated by hecatombs of the slain; His claim is that of having multiplied the human race and happily invoked the Goddess of Health to arrest the arm that scatters pestilence and death over creation."[43] That long awaited day was here and now.

The dread and fear of humanity over the centuries can explain such a joyous outpouring. Meanwhile Jenner pressed forward discussing a smallpox epidemic raging in London. "We have the means of stopping this calamity—Why not employ them. We perceive as it were our houses on fire and with buckets in our hands stand idly by gazing at the flames. Would it not be wise in the Legislature to interfere in the cause of suffering humanity?"[44]

* * * * * *

Yellow fever continued to ravage the port cities of America in the summertime with a disastrous mortality. John Lining of Charlestown, South Carolina, had described yellow fever so well that a correct diagnosis could be made, but doctors had no clue regarding its mode of spread and its treatment.[45] In 1793 a severe epidemic spread throughout Philadelphia and everyone of means fled the city including members of congress and the local government. Infected persons developed malaise, high fever and jaundice. Treatment followed the usual theory of cleansing the body by purges, emetics and bleeding.

Copious bleeding was thought to be necessary. Rush believed his cures increased when he accepted the recommendation of Lining to bleed patients liberally. Lining wrote in 1741, "The physician must not falter and deny treatment just because the patient is weak...an ill timed scrupulousness about the weakness of the body..." was to be disregarded. Bleed and purge even with a feeble pulse, even if the bowels were bloody from the evacuations from the jalop and calomel. Most often he recommended bleeding a total of at least sixty ounces and sometimes he bled eighty ounces; usually thirty ounces were bled at one sitting (equivalent to almost two standard transfusion units).[46,47,48]

The epidemic of 1793 is well described in Benjamin Rush's *Letters*. Rush believed that calomel (mercury compound) given with jalop (a dried root) cured the disease. He stated that ninety-nine out of one hundred people who took this medication on the first day of the disease survived. Rush carried on a bitter feud with other doctors in the city who refused to follow his treatment. He personally attacked other physicians who claimed his success was based upon treating patients who did not, in the first place, have the disease. The bitterness among doctors spread to their patients who championed one doctor over another. Rush became increasingly assertive, claiming the other doctors were plotting against him. He went so far as to pay for a bulletin in the *Federal Gazette* in which he addressed the people of Philadelphia, recommending his mercurial purges and criticizing doctors who spoke against his treatment.

This advertisement was rebutted by another printed in the *Gazette of the United States and Advertiser* in 1794, written by Dr. William Currie. Currie pulled no punches in his attack on Rush and in his advertisement stated, "An impartial Review of that part of Dr. Rush's publication on the Yellow Fever which treats of its origin. In which his opinions are shown to be erroneous—the Introduction of the disease by importation proved, and the whole someness of the city vindicated—and at the same time may be had Dr. Curries Treatise on the Yellow Fever and his account of Climates and diseases of America—by Wm. Currie Fellow of the College of Physicians."[49] Currie was right that the disease was imported, but its method of spread remained a mystery. Doctors sparring in public increased the despair among the stricken.

Hysteria gripped the city, and its citizens responded to any suggestions to protect themselves from the disease. *Dunlap's American Daily Advertiser* on August 25, 1793, recommended a "recipe" for preventing infection with yellow fever: "Take of rue, sage, mint, rosemary, wormwood and lavender a handful of each—infuse them together in a gallon of white wine vinegar, put the whole in a stone pot, closely covered up upon warm wood ashes for four days. After straining, the liquid is put in a quart bottle with an ounce of camphor... With this preparation wash your mouth and rub your loins and temples every day, sniff a little up your nostrils when you go into the air and carry about with you a sponge dipped in the same to smell... especially when you are near any place or person that is infected."[50]

Fifty to one hundred people daily were dying of the fever. During one three-month period in 1793, ten percent of the population died. In spite of complete lack of knowledge of the causes of this disease and the futility of the treatment, we must admire Rush and the other physicians who stayed in the city, exposing themselves to the disease daily, not knowing who amongst them would succumb next. Three of Rush's apprentices died of the disease and Rush describes getting three or four hours of sleep each day and often having to refuse fifty patients a day for lack of time.[51]

With the cooler weather of fall, the disease abated. It was more than one hundred years later before the mosquito was shown to be the vector of this malady.

* * * * * *

The first appearance of venereal disease in the Massachusetts Bay Colony was described by Governor John Winthrop in 1646. "There fell out also a bothersome disease at Boston which raised a scandal upon the town and country though without just cause. One, of the town _____ having gone cooper on a ship; at his return his wife was infected with Lues Venereum which appeared thus: being delivered of a child and nothing then appearing, but the midwife, a skillful woman finding the body as sound as any other after her delivery, she had a sore breast whereas divers neighbors resorting to her, some of them drew her breast, and other suffered their children to draw her and others, let her child suck them (no such disease being suspected by any), by occasion about 16 people, men, women, and children were infected whereby it came at length to be discovered by such in the town that had skill in physic and surgery, but there was not any in the country who had been practiced in that cure.... And it was observed that many did eat and drink and lodge in bed with those infected and had sores, yet none of them took it of them but by copulation or sucking."[52]

Governor Winthrop proved to be a good epidemiologist and recognized a venereal transmission, but it was more likely another venereal disease than syphilis.

The venereal transmission of syphilis was known and it was one of the diseases in which a cure was thought possible by use of calomel. In reality there is a long remission between the secondary and tertiary stages of syphilis, which acts on the vascular and central nervous systems. It is likely that the tertiary symptoms were not thought to be related to syphilis.

John Hunter, in London, wondered about the origin of venereal disease. It is not found in animals and, according to Hunter, it arose in "modern times"; but where, in America, the West Indies, Europe? Hunter knew that the first stages of syphilis were seen in the skin; later the bones and tendons were involved. Mercury was thought to be the cure, but it can, itself, cause toxicity such as salivation, headaches and a sallow complexion. Hunter seems to be confused about syphilis and gonorrhea. At times he describes the two diseases as different manifestations of the same malady. He states that venereal disease is a poison, and it includes syphilis and gonorrhea. In the one instance it causes a chancre; in the other, pus. At other times, he states that gonorrhea is time limited and needs only astringents. It is doubtful that Hunter was aware of the later stages of these diseases as they affect the nerves, brain and circulation. In his book, there is no mention of congenital syphilis, and it is doubtful that Hunter or any other physician in this period knew of this aspect of the disease.[53]

Hunter, in what was probably a political maneuver, accused the French for the introduction of gonorrhea into Tahiti. When Captain Cook on his last voyage visited Tahiti, the disease was present, whereas the island was free of it on his previous voyage. Hunter showed that Captain Wallis of England sailed nonstop to Tahiti, leaving Plymouth in August, 1766, and arriving in July, 1767. Over such a long uninterrupted voyage gonorrhea "could not survive." On the other hand, Captain Bougainville left France in December 1766 and arrived after several stops, en route, in April 1768 and, therefore, must be responsible. Moreover, Captain Wallis' crew "was more disciplined".[54]

In Europe the wandering leper with his bell to announce his coming was a common sight in the cities of earlier centuries. It continued to be diagnosed in the eighteenth century, but there is no record of it in America. Canker sore, which has similar symptoms to leprosy, was starkly described by Hamilton in rural England. Hamilton noted that a few children in his practice were seen each year with mild ulceration and inflammation of the gums. The disease progressed inexorably in spite of treatment. After the ulceration, the teeth of the children became rotten and dropped out, following which the jawbone was destroyed. The cartilage of the nose sunk and the remaining bones of the face might then be destroyed. Sometimes leg ulcerations developed. It was noted that each year several children were involved but it could never be called an epidemic. In one case, examination of the mother revealed leprous blotches. Was this leprosy? Much more likely it was congenital syphilis. In America, syphilis was often diagnosed, and congenital syphilis must have been a problem, but it wasn't identified.[55]

* * * * * *

Marsh remittent fever or autumnal bilious fever developed around marshy or swampy areas. Hamilton described his experience with this disease in Suffolk County in England in 1782 and 1783. His patients complained of chilliness, heat, fever, cold extremities, headache and vomiting. All symptoms abated for a few hours and then returned. Recurrent remissions were characteristic of this malady and if it intensified, coma and death occurred. Urine was bloody as was saliva and stools. Hamilton observed this was a poisonous miasma from the marshes which responded to "the bark" (cinchona, bark from which quinine is extracted). Patients also improved, if they moved out of the area.[56] This condition has many of the features of malaria and may be similar to the bilious fever described by Pringle. It was also described in South Carolina.[57]

The problem of sorting out the descriptive maladies of the eighteenth century requires the patient analysis of a detective story. There are usually some features of the disease that don't fit a disease classification according to our present knowledge. When we consider that the unfortunate victim was dehydrated and possibly had secondary conditions, such as scurvy and perhaps a superimposed virus or a bacterial complication, one understands the complexity of diagnosis.

* * * * * *

Consumption caused about one tenth of the deaths in London and was frequently diagnosed in America. The susceptible population was mostly young people between the ages of fifteen and thirty years and were described as having a slender build. Most, but probably not all of these cases, had pulmonary tuberculosis. Not being epidemic, its infectious nature was never emphasized, but some physicians advised children against being close to a consumptive patient. Though it was frequently diagnosed in America, it was thought to be more prevalent in Britain than anywhere in the world.

To avoid it, exercise and fresh air were advised. Cold, humid air and violent passions were to be avoided. The symptoms looked for by the physician were a dry cough, hectic fever, night sweats, pain on breathing, spitting of blood and a flushed face. When patients were far gone with this distemper, they appeared ghastly, like "stalking ghosts". Treatment at that time and for the next 175 years, until the discovery of an effective antibiotic (Streptomycin), was country air, exercises, and a wholesome diet, added to which the eighteenth-century physician prescribed woman's milk sucked from the breast.[58]

* * * * * *

Throat distemper appeared epidemically in America. It was also called the "child's plague" and was known to be epidemic. The swollen throat made swallowing and breathing difficult. Later a white coating lined the throat, turning black as the child struggled to breathe.[59] One recorded epidemic occurred in May 1735 in Kingston, New Hampshire, and was again ascribed to bad air. It rapidly spread throughout New Hampshire and northwest Massachusetts, exacting its greatest toll on children and sometimes causing the death of three or more children in a single family. In Haverhill, more than half of the children died and twenty-three families were left childless. The epidemic spread of the disease moved many in the community to isolate the affected. It was thought that the children contracted the disease huddled about the fire in the one-room schoolhouse during winter months. The Reverend Joseph Emerson castigated his parishioners for isolation of the ill. "It is an inordinate and sinful fear that you have of this distemper, if it keeps you from going nigh your neighbors to tend to them and watch with them, or in any other respect to be helpful to them." It drove the people to the churches for prayer and meditation and fast days were proclaimed. "How terrible hath God been in his doings."[60] The disease never got a foothold in Boston because, as Boston physicians proudly proclaimed, they were more effective in curing it. In all probability, Boston citizens had been exposed to diphtheria over a long time period and no pool of susceptible people was available.

Samuel Bard, professor of medicine in Kings' College in New York, wrote about diphtheria which he called "Angina Suffocativa", describing a family with seven children, all of whom contracted the disease and three of whom died. He did postmortem examinations on some of the children and showed that death resulted from mucous and thickening of the membranes of the throat and trachea, which caused suffocation. He did not attribute the cause to toxic air, but an "effluvia" from the breath passed form person to person. Treatment followed the usual remedies.[61]

* * * * * *

Fothergill in London described angina pectoris. His studies came breathtakingly close to the true pathology of this condition. He described several of his patients developing "severe spasmodic chest pain" when walking up a hill or against the wind. He was

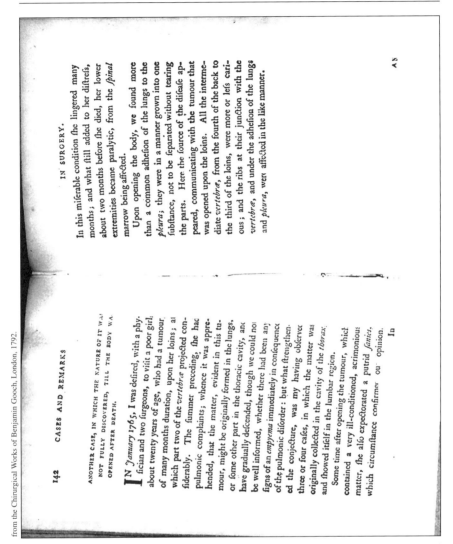

from the Chirurgical Works of Benjamin Gooch, London, 1792.

The Puzzle of Tuberculosis. Benjamin Gooch, surgeon in England, identifies a series of linked symptoms which he correctly diagnosed as starting in the lung, spreading to the spine, causing paralysis and draining pus in the groin.

CASES AND REMARKS

ANOTHER CASE, IN WHICH THE NATURE OF IT WAS NOT FULLY DISCOVERED, TILL THE BODY WAS OPENED AFTER DEATH.

In January 1765, I was defired, with a phyfician and two furgeons, to vifit a poor girl, about twenty years of age, who had a tumour of many months duration, upon her loins; at which part two of the *vertebrae* projected confiderably. The fummer preceding, fhe had pulmonic complaints; whence it was apprehended, that the matter, evident in this tomour, might be originally formed in the lungs, or fome other part in the thoracic cavity, and have gradually defcended, though we could not be well informed, whether there had been any figns of an *empyema* immediately in confequence of the pulmonic diforder: but what strengthened the conjecture, was my having obferved three or four cafes, in which the matter was originally collected in the cavity of the *thorax* and fhowed itfelf in the lumbar region.

Some time after opening the tumour, which contained a very ill-conditioned, acrimonious matter, fhe alfo expectorated a putrid *faries* which circumftance confirmed our opinion.

IN SURGERY

In this miferable condition fhe lingered many months; and what *ftill* added to her diftrefs, about two months before fhe died, her lower extremities became paralytic, from the *fpinal* marrow being affected.

Upon opening the body, we found more than a common adhefion of the lungs to the *pleura*; they were in a manner grown into one fubftance, not to be feparated without tearing the parts. Here the fource of the difeafe appeared, communicating with the tumour that was opened upon the loins. All the intermediate *vertebra*, from the fourth of the back to the third of the loins, were more of lefs carious; and the ribs at their junction with the *verte-bra*, and under the adhefion of the lungs and *pleura*, were affected in the like manner.

perplexed about the origin of the complaint. Did it arise from a disturbance of the lungs or throat or the chest wall or perhaps the heart? One of his patients described a stricture surrounding his chest... "in such a manner to render it impossible to take a step without the hazard of immediate suffocation." He described radiation of pain to the arms in this patient. Could it be due to irritation of the nerves? He sought for the tiniest of clues to find the seat of the problem. The patient suddenly died after a fit of rage.

Fothergill requested John Hunter, the expert anatomist and teacher, to examine the body. Hunter did a thorough autopsy and reported the lungs, chest wall, and throat to be normal. Hunter stated,

"The heart to external appearance was also sound...but upon examination, I found that the substance was paler than common...and in
many parts of the left ventricle it was almost white, having just the
appearance of a beginning ossification. The two coronary arteries from
their origin to their many ramifications upon the heart were become
one piece of bone."

Without a microscope he had no way to identify the sclerotic
plaques impregnated with calcium. The link between the patency of
the coronary arteries and the scars in the heart escaped both Fothergill
and Hunter. The missing part of the puzzle describing the dynamics
of angina pectoris and coronary artery heart disease would be made
more than a hundred years later.[62]

* * * * * *

Much of the medical literature of this century concerns the bites of
rabid animals and the incidence of death from this cause must have
been large.

The full course of development of symptoms following the bite of
a rabid dog is described in a handwritten book covering all diseases
and injuries, one page in English and the opposing page in German,
presumably in use in German-speaking communities of
Pennsylvania.[63]

"For the Bite of a mad dog, when a person is bit by Such
a Dog, the Wound commonly heals up as readily as if it
was not in the least Poisonous. But after the Expiration of
a Longer or Shorter Term from 3 weeks to 3 months, But
most commonly in 6 weeks, the Person bitten Begins to
perceive In the spot that was bit A Certain Dull obtuse
pain. The Scar of it swells Inflames bursts open and
weeps out a Sharp Foetid and serous somewhat bloody

humour, at the same time the Patient becomes sad and melancholic. He feels a kind of indifference and general numbness and almost incessant Coldness, A Difficulty of breathing and continual anguish and pain in the bowels...the madness is attended with the following symptoms, the patient is afflicted with a violent thirst and pain on drinking. Soon after this he avoids all drink...the horror becomes so violent that the bringing of water near his lips or into his sight....affects him with extreme anguish or convulsions."

And then the simple concluding sentence,...

"There is no cure."

In England, Fothergill was more optimistic.

"Mr. Charles Bellany of Holborn, aged forty years on the 14th of February 1774, was bit by a cat which was rabid the same morning. A servant maid was bit in the leg by the same cat just before her master. Both took a recommended remedy. About the middle of April, he complained of pain in the right knee which he supposed was the rheumatism. ....he was prescribed some medication. On Thursday the 16 of June he sent for me, complaining of having had a restless night and told me he had eat some bread and butter as usual for breakfast, yet he found he could not swallow his tea without difficulty. He attempted it before me and threw a little in his mouth but with the utmost agitation."

The above record was written to Fothergill by W. French, an apothecary treating Mr. Bellany to this point, who recognized the symptoms of rabies and called Fothergill to continue treatment. Fothergill noted that the patient swallowed tea with difficulty, but could eat moistened bread. The patient had forgotten about the bite of the cat and Fothergill carefully avoided bringing it back to his memory, but did discuss the entire matter with the family and requested a consultation. Fothergill wrote:

> "The following day his countenance bespoke much distress although accompanied with endeavors to conceal it....He had now a copious flow of saliva.... Warm baths provided him with 'joyous relief'. Many medication were given and he was bled. A vast quantity of phlegm kept collecting in his mouth and he expired forcefully to get rid of all the phlegm. This occasioned a sound which did not seem very remote from the hollow barking of a dog. The patient described his aversion to water as 'hydrophobia' yet without giving any reason he had the slightest idea he was suffering from the disease. Later he became delirious and expired quietly. Before death the bite was not carefully examined for fear of alarming the patient. After death it was minutely examined but it was healed and without evidence of inflammation."

The master's wound healed, but the servant's did not and taxed the skill of a young surgeon who couldn't get it to heal. The young woman was sent to the hospital and was lost to follow-up, but Fothergill had good reason to believe she survived.

Fothergill remarked that a study of this case was an argument for enlarging the wound made by a rabid animal and irritating the wound so it would not heal. He also recommended that suspected animals not be killed so one could observe if they turned mad and died.[64]

* * * * * *

Among all the medicines available to the Colonial doctor, only two have survived into the era of scientific medicine. Peruvian bark or quinine was used for malaria, but without any knowledge of its action, and it was also used to reduce a fever and for relief of pain. It was the 'aspirin' of that period. Laudanum, or opium, was also widely used to relieve pain and was also used in surgery to substitute for an anesthetic.

Mercury was employed for many conditions, particularly syphilis, but it was only partially effective. William Heberden of London, at the conclusion of a long career practicing medicine, stated that of all the remedies he prescribed only five could be relied on: Peruvian bark for the agues, quicksilver (mercury) for venereal disease, sulfur for the itch, opium for the spasms, and Bath waters for the stomach pain caused by drinking. "The above are proven remedies."[65]

The physician was handicapped in treating an ill patient without knowledge of the cause of the illness. His prescriptions used a large number of substances, often six or more, and he was ignorant of which were effective and which were not. Add to this the protracted course of the disease and the many complications that could occur, so that he was treating a complex of conditions. He was rarely in a position when he could separate one disease from another. The predicament of Dr. John Jones treating Benjamin Franklin without a specific diagnosis and without effective medication is a study in frustration. Dr. John Jones attended Benjamin Franklin at his death and gives us a lucid description of a learned physician studying and seeking to comprehend the disease process of his patient. He notes the progression of symptoms, but is helpless to act.

"The stone with which he had been afflicted for several

years had for the last twelve months of his life confined him chiefly to bed; and during the extremely painful paroxysms, he was obliged to take large doses of laudanum to mitigate his tortures; still in the intervals of pain he not only amused himself by reading and conversing cheerfully with his family and a few friends who visited him, but was often employed in doing business of a public as well as a private nature with various persons who waited upon him for that purpose; and in every instance displayed not only the readiness and disposition to do good, which were the distinguishing characteristics of his life, but the fullest and clearest possession of his uncommon abilities. He also not infrequently indulged in those 'jeu d'esprit' and entertaining anecdotes which were the delight of all who heard them.

About sixteen days before his death a fever disposition without any particular symptoms attending it till the third or fourth day, when he complained of pain in his left breast which increased until it became extremely acute, attended by cough and laborious breathing. During this state, when the severity of his pain drew forth a groan of complaint he would observe he was afraid he did not bear them as he ought; acknowledging his grateful sense of the many blessings he had received from the Superior Being who has raised him from small and low beginnings to such high rank and consideration among men; and made no doubt but that his present affliction were kindly intended to wean him from a world in which he was no longer fit to act the part assigned to him. In this frame of body and mind he continued until five days before his death, when the pain and difficulty of breathing left him entirely and his family were flattering themselves with the hope of his recovery; but an imposthume (abscess) which had opened in his lung suddenly burst and discharged a quantity of matter which he continued to throw up while he had the power, but as that failed, the organs of respiration became gradually oppressed; a calm lethargic state succeeded and on the seventeenth inst. (April, 1790) at eleven o'clock at night he expired closing a long and useful life of eighty-four years and three months.

It may not be amiss to the above account that Dr. Franklin, in the year 1734, had a severe pleurisy which terminated in an abscess of his lung and he was then almost suffocated by the quantity and suddenness of the discharge. A second attack of a similar nature happened some years later from which he soon recovered; and he did not appear to suffer any inconvenience in his respiration from these diseases."[66]

Doctors of present day medical science can consider the differential diagnosis leading to the death of Dr. Franklin from this detailed report.

A little over a year later in June, 1791, Jones rode out on horseback to make a medical visit to Charles Thomson, former secretary of the Continental Congress, and returned home exhausted. Several days later on June 17, 1791, he made a visit to Washington and visited several other patients as he returned home. His asthma recurred, followed by other symptoms and he died on June 22, 1791.

* * * * * *

Washington was treated by Dr. James Craik, a long-time friend and neighbor at Mount Vernon who had been born in Scotland and attended the School of Medicine at Edinburgh. Dr. Cullen, on the staff at Edinburgh, had described a disease of the throat, "Cynanche Trachealis." Washington's death, unlike Franklin's, was sudden and unexpected and diagnosed by Craik as "Cynanche Trachealis."

On the twelfth of December 1799, Washington inspected his farm; a cold wind was driving a mixture of snow, rain and hail. The following morning he complained of a sore throat and hoarseness. Colonel Lear, who was with him, suggested he take some medicine to which the general replied he never took anything to carry off a cold, but let it go as it came. The following day, Saturday, December fourteenth, he was taken with a fever and his throat became more sore. Still resistant to call his friend and neighbor Dr. Craik, he asked his overseer to bleed him and 12 ounces of blood were removed from his arm. Washington thought this was not enough and later in the day he called Dr. Craik. Dr. Dick, another neighbor, was also present.[67,68]

Breathing, speaking and swallowing were difficult and painful and Craik prescribed antimony and calomel as medication, and also applied heated cups to blister the skin and draw out the disease as well as vinegar vapors to be inhaled to ease the breathing. Again he was bled; this time 32 ounces was said to have been removed. Breathing became more and more difficult and he died between 10 and 11 p.m. on Saturday night, December 14, 1799.

Dr. John Archer in 1798 wrote a dissertation on cynanche trachealis, also termed acute asthma, catarrh, or suffocative croup. According to Archer it most often affects children often many children in the same family, with symptoms of fever, hoarseness, and cough sometimes associated with a skin eruption. The mechanical obstruction to breathing produces a cough "...so shrill that I can compare it to nothing more than a note emitted from a highly toned instrument." The problem was thought to be the foreign membrane in the throat which impedes breathing so that the patient dies in two or three days of suffocation.[69] Archer was probably describing diphtheria which in common with Washington's symptoms obstructed the air passages, but in Washington's disease it was more likely an acute laryngitis and bronchitis, perhaps caused by a streptococcus infection. A tracheotomy, an incision in the neck opening into the trachea, was described in the eighteenth century, but rarely performed. Perhaps it could have been life saving.

Craik has been accused of excessive bleeding of Washington. If 44 ounces of blood were removed, that would represent over 25% of the average total blood volume. Yet John Lining and Benjamin Rush, prominent American physicians in this period, recommended 60 ounces of bleeding and occasionally 80 ounces. When it was rumored shortly after Washington's death that Craik removed 32 ounces of blood, he denied it.[70]

In 1860, sixty-one years later, Dr. James Jackson reviewed the treatment of Washington by Craik and vigorously upheld treatment by bleeding and medication. Jackson concluded that in 1860 the diagnosis would be acute aryngitis, a swelling of the lining of the windpipe which was so severe it was "in fact strangulation as much as if a tight cord had been twisted around his neck." Jackson said Craik's treatment could not be faulted and that the bleeding was intended to reduce the swollen membranes.[71]

* * * * * *

Seafaring was an important part of national life, both in the American colonies as well as in the mother country. Ships crossed the Atlantic carrying on a brisk trade of cotton, tobacco, lumber and furs eastward and returning with manufactured goods to the ports of Charleston, the Virginia Tidewater, Baltimore, Philadelphia, New York and Boston. American-built ships were busy in coastal trading as well as in the West Indies. During the Colonial period, Britain fought naval battles against Holland, France and Spain, and American seamen with or without their consent manned many of the warships leaving American ports. With the outbreak of the war, the American maritime tradition gained renewed energy, and voyages were made to France, Holland, and the West Indies seeking war material and providing the goods at home normally supplied by Britain. American warships and privateers preyed upon British shipping and remained at sea for long periods, their crews enduring scurvy and the medical hardships of long sea voyages as well as the dangers of naval warfare.

In 1593, on a voyage from England to Chile, Richard Hawkins wrote about the misery and the diseases suffered by his crew of which about one half were affected with scurvy. Hawkins wrote, "And I wish that some learned man would write of it, for it is the plague of the sea and the spoyle of mariners; doubtlesse it would be a worke worthy of a worthy man and most beneficiall for our countries, for in twenty yeeres since I have used the sea I dare take upon me, to give account of ten thousand men consumed with this disease."[72]

Even before Hawkins, we have reference to scurvy. John Woodall, born in 1569, wrote a book for young naval surgeons, *The Surgeons Mate*. There is a section of the book devoted to scurvy which Woodall thought was a disease of the spleen due to a prolonged diet of salt provisions, want of cleanliness and change of clothing. He described the symptoms of the disease precisely and, remarkably, suggested the juice of lemons to provide an extraordinary cure. If lemons were not available, acid vegetable juices were to be used. Moreover, he did not relate the disease to lack of pure air, the explanation of the cause cited in the eighteenth century.[73] With improved navigation, the age of exploration drew ships to all parts of the world on longer and longer voyages, but scurvy decimated crews and foiled many an adventurous effort. In the first voyage of the East India Company in the early seventeenth century, rounding the Cape of Good Hope en route to India, 105 men of a crew of 480 died of scurvy. Lord Anson, attempting to circumnavigate the globe, lost so many men from scurvy that he had to abandon two of his ships to man a third. Yet Captain Cook in 1770 completed a three-year trip around the world between latitudes of 52 degrees north to 72 degrees south and lost only one man of a crew of 118. Cook made frequent and prolonged landings, allowing his crew to stock up on fresh supplies.[74]

Hawkins had good reason to hope someone could cure the ravages of the disease exacted on his crews. Scorbutic crews developed livid spots on the skin, blotches from hemorrhage from nothing more than touching the skin or a minor bump. This was followed by bloating and excessive salivation, bleeding gums, and teeth falling out; an offensive odor surrounded the victim; finally, an anxiety state, lassitude, weakness so severe that walking was impossible, fainting, and loss of consciousness until death blessedly came.

James Lind, surgeon in the British navy in the mid-eighteenth century, is most closely associated with treatment of the scorbutic sailor. But Lind didn't recognize the disease as a dietary deficiency.

In his essay on "The Most Effectual Means of Preserving the Health of Seamen," in 1757, Lind concluded that scurvy was caused by failure of the pores to open and to allow body poisons to escape. The cause was overcrowding and toxic air with bad ventilation below decks and uncleanness which generated a corrupted blood and a putrid fever which was contagious and spread throughout the crew. Although Lind had an imaginative concept of the cause, he knew what the treatment should be: green vegetables or fresh fruit opened the closed pores.[75]

Lind, in his essay on the health of seamen, states regarding scurvy that clean air is necessary to prevent this distemper, but the mischief sometimes lurked in the tainted apparel and filth and rags of impressed seamen. He describes an event of toxic air escaping from the rags of prisoners being tried in court in Newgate which infected and killed the judges hearing their case. To avoid this situation on shipboard, Lind recommended to the admiralty that all impressed sailors and those picked up in prisons and on the streets be sent to a holding area where their clothes would be burned, cleansing accomplished, and fresh clothing supplied before boarding their assigned ships. In this case, Lind was describing typhus transferred by the body louse.

Newly constructed ships were thought to emanate vapors of toxic air from the green timbers. To decontaminate the air, fires were lighted between decks and fed with resin or pieces of tarred rope. Once scurvy developed fresh vegetables and fruit were the best treatment. In northern climates where scurvy is caused by suppressed respiration, garlic, onions, shallots, and leeks opened up the pores. Vegetables, particularly watercress, can be grown from seed on a wet blanket set out on deck to provide oxygenated fresh food.

Thomas Beddoes wrote a book on scurvy, republished in 1797 in Philadelphia, in which he argued that lack of oxygen was the responsible culprit. Food must contain adequate amounts of oxygen to offset the disease. He described some members of crews who when visiting distant ports bartered their food allowances with the natives for local food and thus did not contract the disease. Freshly grown food, he maintained, contained lots of oxygen.

Beddoes described the disease among slaves brought from Africa to America who were overcrowded below decks and without sufficient oxygen. They were stowed below "spoonwise" so close together that they were locked into one another's arms. The rooms were never aired and the temperature was over 96°. Captain Cook, he relates, avoided scurvy on his long voyages by keeping his ships well aired.[76]

Dr. Trotter was quoted by Beddoes as having the ridiculous notion that the disease was due to lack of green vegetables alone and not due to lack of oxygen. Trotter rejected the theories of Lind and Beddoes and insisted that the disease was due to a faulty diet, not toxic air. He recommended less salted meat and more vegetables.

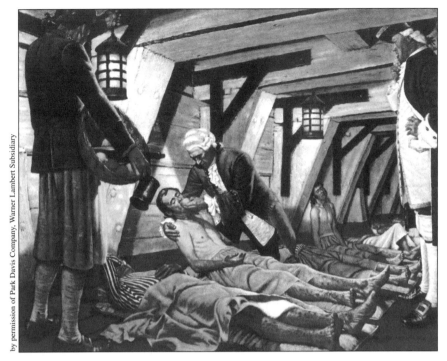

by permission of Park Davis Company, Warner Lambert Subsidiary

JAMES LIND: CONQUEROR OF SCURVY
Surgeon of Britain's Royal Navy abroad H.M.S. Salisbury, in English Channel in 1747. James Lind conducted a series of clinical experiments that definitely proved citrus fruits or their juices would cure scurvy, the dreaded dietary-deficiency disease that killed a million seamen between 1600 and 1800. Dr. Lind's work, at sea, in Edinburgh, and at Haslar Naval Hospital, plus his three books, on scurvy, on care of sailors' health, and on tropical diseases, had much to do with reforming naval health practices, saving lives both on sea and land, and shaping destinations of nations, as world commerce increased.

Moreover he distrusted evaporated juices because the heat destroyed some of the benefit of the fresh fruits and vegetables. He described lemon juice put into quart bottles, protected by a layer of olive oil and securely stoppered to exclude air and stored in a cool place on board ship. He described treating some scorbutic slaves on board a slave ship plying between Guinea in the African Coast to the West Indies who recovered with treatment of this juice after it had been stored fourteen months.

Trotter had a strong social conscience and was critical of the admiralty describing the horrors of impressment. How could they kidnap a seaman going home to his friends and family after a long voyage, and then force him aboard another ship about to sail for a several month journey? He was an experienced naval surgeon, frequently traveling on slave ships which often had a cargo of 300 to 400 slaves. He noted their illnesses, and made practical suggestions about their diet including fresh fruit syrup. He advised the captains to allow the slaves on deck daily, teaching them to cleanse themselves while the dark holds in which they were stored were cleaned. All those not regarded as dangerous should be freed of leg and arm irons. For exercise he advised allowing them "to be danced to the sound of drums while on deck of which they are very fond..." wind foils were to be used to provide below deck ventilation.[77]

Later in the eighteenth century, citrus fruits were recognized for their ability to prevent and cure scurvy, and instructions for concentrating juice that would survive a long journey are described. "Pour the juice into a vessel and gently heat over a fire but prevent boiling. Concentrate until it is a thick syrup and put the syrup in bottles." Each crew member received a few drops of the syrup mixed with water daily. Twenty-five pounds of oranges would yield five ounces of syrup.[78]

* * * * * *

With the ending of the Revolutionary War, some medical advances were made. The first census authorized by Congress in 1790 counted 3,928,326 inhabitants; by 1800 the number had swelled to 5,319,762. By 1800 there were 250 medical school graduates from the University of Pennsylvania in Philadelphia, College of Physicians and Surgeons in New York, Dartmouth in New Hampshire and Harvard at Boston. Most physicians still were trained as apprentices. There was one doctor for 800 people in the cities and one for ten to twelve thousand in the rural areas.

Doctors' fees were low. John Archer, of the first medical school class of the College of Philadelphia, practiced for a period in Delaware. His fee schedule was 2 shillings, 6 pence for bleeding; £1 for a smallpox inoculation; 2 shillings, 6 for a tooth extraction; a home visit was 5 shillings and 1 shilling was to be charged for every mile over five miles; night calls were 10 shillings.[79] During the war, Jonathan Potts, practicing in Lancaster, Pennsylvania, recorded charging 1 to 5 shillings for a visit depending on its length; an extra shilling was charged for a night call. To fix a broken finger, the cost was 15 shillings; £1 to reduce an elbow and £2 for a fracture of the thigh.[80] John Syng Dorsey's daybook records 260 patients in July 1808 and he received an annual cash income of $1,734.00.[81]

CHAPTER TWO

SURGICAL PRACTICE

Surgery, in Colonial times, was concerned with the repair of the physical damage to an involved part and treatment was dictated by the body part itself and the extent of the damage. Some surgeons did elective operations, but most surgery was reparative. In contrast to the difficulty in making a diagnosis in medicine, the diagnosis in surgery was usually more easily made, particularly after injuries. The lacerations caused by a blow of the sword exposed the structures to be repaired. A penetrating wound of a dagger, lance, arrow, bayonet or a musket ball often follows a straight line path and a precise knowledge of anatomy would suggest which structures would be damaged in the course of the penetrating metal. The diagnosis being evident, the treatment was simplified. Those doctors who studied in a medical school had the opportunity to dissect and study human anatomy and were expert anatomists. Those who were certified by apprenticeship often learned their anatomy from textbooks and some apprentices had opportunities to attend anatomical lectures and demonstrations.

Thus, no elaborate theory need be invoked such as was true in medicine. Restore the damaged structures to normal. Moreover, the alert surgeon could inspect the wound from day to day and compare its progress with what he knew to be a benign healing course. Being able to visually inspect and follow the course of a wound, he quickly learned what treatment promoted healing and which treatment delayed healing. Each wounded patient was a learning experience. Did the wound drain pus locally as expected? Was there undue spreading of the wound or swelling and redness or retained pus? Different types of treatment could be compared by following the healing process. Those that lead to a favorable result were described in reports, those that failed were discarded. The patient lived or died, or survived with a disability. This was the ultimate test of a treatment. This empirical knowledge was passed along from century to century and a formidable body of surgical knowledge preserved.

The role of the surgeon was constrained to controlling hemorrhage, treatment of wounds, repairing muscles and tendons, and reducing dislocations and fractures. When faced with abdominal wounds, he restricted his efforts to repacking exposed viscera and closure of the wound. If he could identify a bleeding vessel proximal to the wound, he would attempt to control the bleeding; but he was wary of entering the abdominal cavity and repair of the abdominal contents. Perhaps his caution was because he recognized the unavoidable complication of peritonitis and death. Some patients with abdominal wounds survived, but mostly they were written off as beyond hope. Except on rare occasions, he avoided the chest as beyond his scope, but there are reports of patients shot in the chest who lived. Removal of air from the chest cavity, in particular air under pressure, is such a dramatic and life-saving procedure, it is surprising that no mention of it is made in surgical texts.

James Thacher described a wound of the lungs and shoulder treated by a Doctor Eustis. Air escaped at every breath. Eustis repeatedly bled the soldier, almost to death, on the theory that the more desperate the circumstances, the more you should bleed. No attempt was made to seal the wound so air would not escape, but the patient was reported as recovering.[82] These areas were off limits, and so was the cranial cavity, except for trephination or the making of drill holes in the skull.

Surgical elective operations were not done often. However, textbooks describe excision of large tumors near the skin surface and removal of cataracts from the eyes. Frequent operations involved removal of stones from the bladder and repair of herniae.[83]

In each century, pioneer operations of an experimental type were practiced by imaginative surgeons, but they were not often included in the surgical practice of the average doctor. We can trace this restrictive surgical practice to two unyielding gaps in knowledge. The first factor was the lack of an anesthetic agent, permitting detailed unhurried procedures, which limited the surgeon to a rapid slashing wound entrance and a few minutes of closure.

Laudanum or opium was freely used as well as whiskey or rum to reduce pain, which may have made the patient unreasonable and difficult to control. Peruvian bark or quinine was also used to allay pain, but this could be no more effective than an aspirin.

For amputations, a tourniquet was usually used and if the tourniquet was tightly applied and remained in place for more than a few minutes the superficial nerves would fail to conduct and the numbing effect would help to overcome pain, but this would not provide relief when the deeper structures were severed. The tourniquet of course could not be used for operations on the trunk, head, or high in the extremities.

The patient could be provided with cotton to stuff in his ears to keep out the sounds of the saw and other instruments. Many patients probably lost consciousness from reduced blood pressure and bleeding. The application of leeches to the wound edges after surgery to reduce swelling and pain by drawing out fluid was also used. Recent biochemical studies have shown that leeches secrete an anticoagulant known as hirudon, which may provide some pain relief in addition to reducing swelling. Modern surgery has revived the use of leeches to reduce swelling from venous congestion after replacing a severed part.

The second factor was ignorance of the microscopic world of bacteria. Some wounds healed well, while some were infected and patients died of sepsis. Without knowledge of the cause of infection, wound healing was a gamble. Healing was attributed to many other causes, but in truth the die was cast as soon as the wound occurred and depended upon the number and virulence of the bacteria entering it. A few surgeons regarded cleanliness as important and went so far as to wash their hands and carefully wash their instruments; some even poured wine or vinegar on the dressings, both of which are antiseptics.

By the eighteenth century, medicine and surgery had made small advances, but medicine awaited the germ theory of disease and was still strangled by fanciful theories applicable to all diseases and a large pharmacopoeia of impotent, useless, sometimes harmful drugs, while surgery awaited advances in pain control and knowledge of bacteria.

The thought of the pain a patient must endure during an operation without anesthesia makes us recoil. Stoicism in heroic measures is called for to submit to an amputation or trephination (removal of a segment of the skull) and the many other operations which are recorded in this period. Unnecessary operations and operative procedures without good cause were not often recommended. When the patient reached a critical state, the operation became a necessity and the patient agreed. Rarely, the patient could be coerced into an operation by the surgeon.

Dr. Silvester Gardiner was a well-known Boston physician and John Hartshorn was his apprentice, who wrote a detailed report on a patient whose leg was amputated under the title *Tucker's Wife's Leg*. Hartshorn was asked to dress an ulcer of the leg of Mrs. Tucker, daily.

When the ulcer worsened, Hartshorn called the master who decided an operation was necessary.[84] On May 29, 1752, Hartshorn wrote the operative note.

> "Doctor Thos. Williams, Docts. Pecker, Jepson and myself went and amputated Tucker's Wife's leg after much persuasion and many arguments. We sat her in a chair and put a Large Bowl of Sand under her and applyd the tourniquet with a compress or two upon the arteries. I handed the instruments. Dr. Williams held the tourniquet after binding a tape around the leg about five inches below the patella for a Guide to the Knife. D. G. began the incision and divided quite thro the membrane adiposa, then Pecker drawing the skin taut, next the muscles were divided, then the Catlin* to divide the interosseous muscles, then with the saw the leg was separated, five vessels taken up, lint applyd and two pledgets digest over them, two longitudinal pledgets, three double headed bandages, afterwards an anodyne of Batm...brought the leg home and Pecker dissected it."

The patient did well.

In this detailed account, no mention is made of the pain suffered by Mrs. Tucker at surgery or postoperatively. Prior to surgery the surgeons persuaded and argued the patient into having the operation—no voluntary informed consent here.

Surgical texts of this era gloss over the problem of pain during surgery and notes of case reports by surgeons rarely mention pain, yet they must have been affected by the cries of their patients and their writhings, controlled by the brute strength of those restraining the patient.

---

* Catlin — double-edged amputation knife.

Some surgery done in this period involved complicated surgical approaches. To operate quickly in order to reduce the pain and blood loss was mandatory and the surgeons were expert anatomists who knew their way around body structures and took pride in approaching the anatomic site in minutes. Lisfranc, the French surgeon, practicing on cadavers, boasted he could disarticulate a hip in ten seconds. Benjamin Bell in Edinburgh could perform a thigh amputation (all but the bone) in six seconds. Any competent surgeon could perform an amputation in 30 seconds and complete the procedure in three minutes. Such a short operating time seems incredible and some boastful competition can be inferred![85]

* * * * * *

The principles of treatment of wounds and injuries as practiced by the Colonial surgeon two hundred years ago in many ways resembles the treatment of today. The wounding missile, bullet or arrow, almost always must be removed, pus under pressure must be released; an actively draining wound is never closed, but the surgeons could recognize a benign wound and proceed to close it with adhesive plasters or stitches. The details of treatment have, of course, changed.[86]

Even without radiographs the surgeon knew when fractured bones were aligned satisfactorily. When the limbs were of equal length and symmetrical, and matched each other, the fracture was well set.

Problems presenting to the surgeon, then and now, are often mechanical and urgent. This is especially true in regard to injuries. The control of bleeding, restoration and healing of wounds, and bone continuity present the same problems to present-day surgeons that they presented to the Colonial surgeons. Methods at the disposal of modern surgeons are infinitely greater but the principles of treatment coincide.

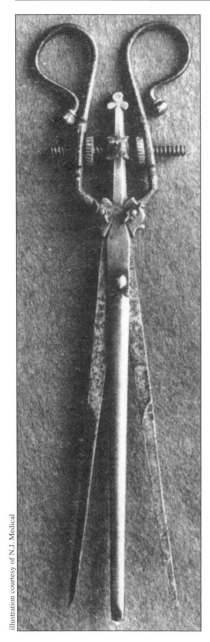

illustration courtesy of N.J. Medical

Arrow extractor from New Jersey Medicine in the Revolutionary era.

Wounds of the skull were trephined to reduce intracranial pressure. Trepanation or trephination as a procedure to cure wounds and ailments of the head, headaches, and sometimes psychiatric behavior, can be traced to ancient man. Skulls with rounded or man-made defects in the cranial vault are often found at archeologic sites. In Colonial times, trephination was the treatment for wounds of the head with depressed bone fragments pressing on the brain, and also was recommended for blunt injuries in patients showing deepening unconsciousness or coma, and was performed with a toothed circular instrument with a handle which was rotated.

Doctor Physick provides a case history of a head injury which he treated.[87,88]

"Michael Schoch, aged about forty, when on the stairs fell backward on the floor; he rose, rubbed his head, and did not suppose himself seriously hurt. About twenty minutes after the accident he felt sick at the stomach and vomited. In one half-hour he became drowsy and stupid, his stupor gradually increasing, and when I saw him which was several hours after the accident, he was perfectly senseless and could not be aroused. His breathing was stertorous, and his pulse, about forty, communicated to the fingers the same sensation as that of a patient in apoplexy.

Upon shaving the head, not the slightest vestige of injury could be observed. From these circumstances, it was very obvious that a blood vessel was ruptured within the cranium. The patient's brother said that he pointed to the left side of his head above the ear after the fall.

And with no other direction than this, I resolved to perforate the parietal bone. Accordingly, I cut through the scalp and applied a trephine; immediately a large quantity of blood escaped and upon passing my fingers under the cranium was literally unable to feel the dura mater. Clots of blood appeared to occupy the whole left hemisphere of the brain...

I determined to make another perforation with the trephine and enlarged the incision.... In a few hours the stupor subsided and the pulse rose.... His right side was slightly paralytic for a few days but no permanent affection of that nature remained."

To perform operations on conscious patients without antisepses or asepses, without devices to fix the part or antibiotics, transfusion of blood, and radiologic control, challenges our imagination and compels us to admire their skill and courage. The fortitude of the patient to submit to a procedure entailing such pain with so uncertain an outcome commands our respect. It contrasts the attitude of people in that century toward life, and their social and religious upbringing with those in modern society. Life was dangerous, death must be faced daily, and the mind was ever ready for its acceptance, with the certain knowledge of a hereafter. The average life span was thirty-five years, the death rate being appalling. In Boston, during that century, the rate was thirty-five people per thousand population each year. Only a very high birthrate allowed the country to grow. The average married woman had seven children.[89]

It is interesting to note that the great subsequent advances that permit the scope of surgery today, for the most part, did not spring from those working in the surgical field but were discoveries in other areas and were introduced into surgery. Such were anesthesia, bacteriology, radiology, blood products, transfusions, and antibiotics.

Infection was the most common cause of death and infection of wounds was the most common condition dealt with by the Colonial surgeon. The shortened life span eliminated much of the cardiac and tumor problems which develop with advancing age and are treated by modern surgeons. Without knowledge of the cause of infection and without effective medication, strong reliance must be placed on the inherent resistance of the patient. When the patient was septic, the surgeon prescribed heat, poultices, fomentations, various impotent drugs and, of course, bleeding. By means of these methods the surgeon hoped for the infection to resolve—that is, for the body's defenses to overcome the infection.

If it failed to resolve and, in particular, if it was accompanied by fever, toxicity and the development of an abscess, release of the pressure forthwith was the accepted treatment. Using an unsterile knife a small incision was made over the abscess and if pus exploded from the incision and the pressure was reduced, a favorable outcome could be expected. The incision was small because the teaching was that the ingress of air was toxic. The toxic air concept was related to their experience in incising clean wounds which developed pus after the surgery. This infection presumably arose from the poisons (bacteria) in the air entering the wound.

If pus continued to collect after incision and drainage was hindered, a curved probe, threaded with candlewick or cotton thread was directed into the incision and perforated the skin at some other point so that the drain hung out at both ends, allowing more complete drainage and preventing the wound from closing.

If the infection did not resolve after these procedures or if the patient was inoperable, recourse to nonsurgical treatment was made and bleeding and medications were continued, but the condition of the patent could be expected to deteriorate as systemic sepsis developed, followed by mortification and death.

Toxicity due to entrance of air into a wound was a widespread concept mentioned in many reports and textbooks.[90] If the skin was breached due to wounding or an incision by the surgeon, signs of infection rapidly developed and it was reasoned that the inrush of air caused the problem. "Air under the skin was like a spark on gunpowder."[91] It was reasoned that the inrush of air caused the problem, and moreover, some types of air were more poisonous than others. The entry of air into a wound as a cause of this problem was so self-explanatory, so convincing, so widespread a theory, that a substance outside the skin, perhaps in the air that could gain entrance into a wound, was not considered.

James Butler was a medical student in Philadelphia who kept a complete notebook of his medical lectures which survives today.[92] In his copybook he has collected notes of Philip Physick and John Dorsey, his professors of surgery. We read of an experiment performed by Physick to test the idea that air was toxic. Air was admitted with a needle into the chest of a kitten and instead of becoming toxic, the kitten suffered no ill effect. Fortunately, infection did not occur or the opposite conclusion would be reached.

The surgeon was called to treat knife and sword wounds as well as bayonet wounds. He was taught to treat hemorrhage by the application of a dressing applied under pressure. If the bleeding vessel was visible, it could be tied with a ligature. If neither of these methods could control the hemorrhage a tourniquet was used whenever possible. If in spite of these measures blood continued to trickle from the wound, the patient might be bled by cutting a vein in his arm. Sufficient blood loss would lower the blood pressure so that the bleeding from the wound slowed to a trickle, dried up and, hopefully, a clot developed over the bleeding vessel so that when the blood pressure again rose, the clot would not be blown out. It was a gamble whether the lowered blood pressure would stop the bleeding before it caused the death of the patient.

Once bleeding was controlled, wounds were not disturbed unless repair of a severed structure was undertaken. Ointments and nostrums of many types were applied, each surgeon having his favorite, but the better-trained surgeons refrained from this practice and simply covered the wound with a dressing. With the cessation of drainage a coverage of dried serum was expected, followed by healing repair tissue.

John Jones, professor of surgery at Kings' College in New York, recommended that fresh wounds be protected from cold and the air by a dry dressing and bandage and advised against ointments.[93] When drainage diminished and the wound had a benign appearance, he would suture the wound or close it with sticking plasters, but no wound was to be closed until after the stage of inflammation.

An alarming complication of any wound, even a very small one was the locked jaw, or tetanus. When faced with this problem, surgeons knew that treatment could only be ameliorative and one hundred percent mortality could be expected. It was common knowledge that small penetrating wounds were most subject to this dreaded complication. All the surgeon could do was to prescribe large doses of opium, warm baths and to maintain a food intake which might require removal of a front tooth to feed the patient through his clamped jaws.[94]

William Cocke wrote a dissertation on tetanus to fulfill his requirement for a doctorate in medicine in Philadelphia in 1798.[95] Cocke describes the development of symptoms of tetanus, beginning with difficulty in swallowing, followed by such severe rigidity of the spinal muscles that the body is arched; supported on the bed by only the head and heels. The spasm is accompanied by severe pain and death occurs in about seven days. Cocke states the condition can sometimes be prevented by incising the associated small wound and instilling stimulants, such as turpentine, to cause inflammation and suppuration. To attempt a cure of the established disease, he emulates the teaching of his professor, Benjamin Rush, prescribing what Rush recommends for all diseases—bleeding, emetics, purgatives and opium.

In his system of surgery, Benjamin Bell of Edinburgh, describing lacerated or contused wounds, recommends that bleeding be first controlled by ligatures, and he describes a modern surgeon's knot, with a double first throw. The limb is then elevated and splinted "in a natural fashion". He cautions not to close the wound. If the patient suffers severe pain, relief can be obtained by fastening leeches to the wound edges. "The wound is dressed with pledgets of lint with an emollient and covered with a warm poultice. If the inflammation (infection) continues, one must be alert for 'mortification' (gangrene)."[96]

The suturing of wounds is mentioned in texts and by many surgeons. John Syng Dorsey, Surgeon of Pennsylvania Hospital, used several pieces of sewing thread twisted together to suture wounds after bleeding was controlled and after washing the wound with warm water.[97] He worried about the effect of inserting any agent foreign to the body and the reaction of the body tissue to this agent.

Catgut and parchment leather were also used. Some surgeons recommended French kid leather cut into one-half-inch strips. The polished part is separated and discarded and the residual strip is wet and stretched. Wounds were also reduced in width by sticking plasters or bandaging.

Philip Syng Physick observed that leather straps used as sutures to bind wounds together dissolved. He went so far as to observe the fate of such sutures placed in a horse. They held, but dissolved later. He tried buckskin parchment, kid leather, and catgut sutures over an ulcer. They all dissolved, but catgut lasted longest. Physick stated, "Future experiments will probably place at the command of the surgeon, a variety of these ligatures which may be so selected as to remain the exact length of time he may require." John Syng Dorsey, nephew of Philip, published the first text by an American author of the entire field of surgery in 1813, where he discussed these experiments.[98]

Bladder stones were removed and occasionally a tumor was removed. Philip Syng Physick, first professor of surgery at the University of Pennsylvania and sometimes known as the father of surgery in the United States, gained fame as an expert lithotomist, operating and removing bladder stones, a condition which at that time seems to have been much more common than encountered today. At the end of his career and in partial retirement, he was asked by Chief Justice of the Supreme Court John Marshall in 1831 to remove his bladder stones. Physick demurred on the basis of his age or perhaps to avoid the anxieties attendant on operating on such a renowned person. He asked Dr. Randolph, trained by him, to do the surgery. Randolph refused and Marshall insisted Physick perform the operation. Over a thousand stones were removed from Marshall's bladder by Physick, who performed a superb technical procedure, and Marshall made a complete recovery. In 1835, when the Chief Justice died, a postmortem examination revealed a normal appearing bladder, without any stones. The postmortem established that he died of an enlarged liver, which was riddled with tuberculous abscesses.

Bell's textbook of surgery observed that a nerve partially cut causes severe pain, which can be relieved by cutting the nerve completely. Since that time, pain from a partially severed nerve has been repeatedly shown to be relieved by completing the severance; or a nerve repair. If a tendon is cut, it will heal if the limb is positioned so the tendon ends are close together and held until secure. It is not necessary to suture the ends as they will unite with scar tissue. If the Achilles tendon is ruptured, a slipper is applied to the foot with the foot held pointed down by the slipper which is tied to the leg and the knee bent to bring the tendon ends together. In two weeks a high-heeled shoe with a strap to the leg is applied.[99]

* * * * * *

FRACTURES

Ed Stafford in London, May 6, 1643, gave a recipe for a broken bone:

> "A broken bone or a joynt dislocated, to knit them: Take ye barke of elm or witch hazzle; cutt away the outward and cutt ye inward redd barke small, and all upon ye Bone or Joynt. Tye it on; and with ye mussilage of it and bole Armeniat make a playster and laye it on—. These receipts are all experimented."[100]

Nicholas Waters, in his text of surgery printed in America, divided fractures into transverse, oblique, longitudinal, compound, or closed.[101] He emphasized the importance of a compound or open fracture. "The smallest external wound communicating with the fracture will be predictive of danger." The difference between an open or closed fracture in today's teaching is still strongly emphasized. In Bell's time, it was the admission of air that was thought to complicate the fracture.

The function of the doctor, Bell explains, is to replace the deranged parts of the bone, bringing the distal part to the proximal part and to retain them in this position as long as necessary and to position the limb so all muscles are relaxed. Thigh and leg fractures will heal in two months, the arm and forearm in six weeks and smaller bones in three weeks. Fractures will heal faster in infancy and childhood. Non-union or failure of the fracture to heal is the result of inadequate support of the fracture, or tendon or muscle interposition, but may also be due to a constitutional disease, such as rickets, scurvy or syphilis.[102]

Again, a discussion of pain during surgery and means to mitigate it, is strangely lacking in discussion of fractures. How many assistants are necessary to restrain the patient and the position of the patient and the surgeon are addressed, but what the patient suffers is not discussed. Bell's book even has a chapter on performing autopsies and embalming; referring to pain, he states that opium is the best narcotic and nerve compression by a tourniquet in amputations diminishes pain.

In his dissertation for the degree of doctor of medicine from the University of Pennsylvania in 1797, Robert Black chose the subject of fractures.[103] The basis for such a dissertation was a full knowledge of the literature extant at the time, plus what little experience he garnered during a very short period in practice. Then, even more than now, different groups advocated methods of treatment which differed and had fiery exchanges advocating their point of view, often on trivial matters. An international controversy divided surgeons: whether a fractured leg should be treated with the knee bent or straight as was customary. The bent knee school was gaining popularity, and its chief advocate was the prestigious Sir Percival Pott in London. Black strongly opposed this principle and wrote his thesis with all the aplomb of a medical student in 1797, or today, who was confident of all the answers and possessed the ultimate knowledge.

In this country, John Jones, professor of Surgery at Kings' College in New York, and a friend of Pott entered the discussion by deriding those surgeons who continued to use the extended position because the increased pain and swelling that resulted made it necessary for the surgeon to cut the dressing and lose position of the bones to relieve such distress.[104] He broadened the argument with a discussion of the types of bandages to be used. He did not approve of long roller bandages because it denied the surgeon access to view the limb, and instead employed an eighteen-tailed bandage over which he placed wood or pasteboard splints secured by leather straps. These could be removed one at a time for inspection of the limb to note the position of the fracture. The bent knee was supported by a pillow and frequently the patient was nursed for the duration in the side-lying position.[105]

Plaster of Paris casts were to enter in the treatment of fractures almost one hundred years later; but Rhazes, an Arabian physician in 860 A.D., used lime mixed with egg white to support a fracture, stating it would become as hard as stone on drying. In Arabia, the development of a firm supportive dressing for a fracture was pursued and Eton, a British consul in Bassora, in his publication, A Survey of the Turkish Empire, written in 1798 stated: "I saw in the eastern part of the Empire a method of setting bones practiced which appears to me worthy of the attention of surgeons in Europe...enclosing a broken limb in a case of plaster of Paris or gypsum which solidifies. If it is too loose, liquid plaster is poured in through a hole in the cast."[106] Credit for the present type of plaster cast is attributed to Matthysen, a medical officer of the Dutch army in 1852. There is no record of the use of a plaster cast in the eighteenth century in Europe or America and all patients with fractures of the lower limbs had to be confined to bed until the fracture healed.

The surgeon manipulated the fracture, applying traction while his assistants held the patient and provided countertraction. The leg was immobilized to allow healing to occur after manual reduction by laying the patient on a board in bed, bandaging the limb with a bulky bandage, perhaps supporting it with pasteboard splints on each side over which the limb was encased in pillows strapped together and wooden shingles were bandaged on either side of the pillows. Final adjustments could be obtained by stuffing rags between the pillow and the limb to correct residual angulation. The ankle and heel are particularly padded. If the fracture was open, the splints must be applied so the wound could be inspected. Sometimes a three-sided fracture box would support the pillow.

The ingenuity of the surgeon was tested in treating fractures of the thigh or femoral shaft, the largest bone in the body surrounded by massive muscles. Most often three long boards—one posteriorly, one medially, and one laterally—extending from the groin to well below the foot were strapped to the padded extremity. Leather straps passed through holes at the end of the splint and looped over the ankle supplied traction. A fracture box also could be employed. These were metal or wooden troughs hinged at the knee, wrapped around the thigh and leg, and tied to an upright fastened to the foot of the bed. After several weeks of traction, it would be released intermittently for exercises to the knee. Position was acceptable when the normal limb matched the fractured one and limb lengths were equal.

Hip fractures were also treated in this way but this fracture was "tedious" in healing, leading to deformity and lameness, and there was little optimism about getting a reduction or union. "The machine was not yet invented to which the thigh bone can be perfectly secured."[107] It still is not invented and must be secured with metal screws today.

The lack of X-ray control and other rigorous standards to assess the final result bred false confidence in the treating surgeon. "Few cases will occur where the surgeon will not be able to get a reduction immediately."[108]

Fractures of the vertebrae were always regarded as fatal. A fracture of the spine was only diagnosed if there was a spinal cord injury and paralysis. Fractures of the spine, not resulting in paralysis, were never diagnosed in the absence of imaging techniques. Occasionally if the wound was open due to a saber cut, the fracture was identified and the surgeon might remove bone fragments pressing on the spinal marrow (cord); in one case reported by Waters, a patient was relieved of his paralysis by this procedure.[109] Fractures with paralysis lead to a slow death due to bowel and bladder dysfunction and sacral sores. Rarely did the patient survive six months.[110]

Most surgeons explained the healing of fractures by the slow flow of a gelatinous marrow toward the break and the solidification of this substance represented the healing of the fracture. John Hunter observed that a blood clot occupied the fracture cavity, not a gelatinous marrow, and he showed that the in-growth of new tissue into this clot were the first phases of a healing fracture. At a later date, Hunter showed cartilage to precede new, solid bone uniting the ends.[111]

If a fracture failed to unite, it lacked a clot or gelatinous matter in the critical area or there was excessive movement of the fracture ends from poor splintage, or perhaps the bone was too badly splintered or too soft to be restored. Muscle tags or tendons might be interposed between the bone ends and prevent healing. The surgeon would diagnose a non-union when the bone ends were still movable, but the patient suffered no pain. Further splintage or immobilization would now be useless. One surgeon asserted that after treating about 1000 fractures, he recalled only five or six "with want of union".[112]

The more courageous surgeons treated a non-union of a closed fracture by incising down to the fracture and removing a small portion of the ends of the bone, freshening the wound to encourage

bleeding, rubbing the ends together and allowing some limited movement of the fracture so the ends would continue to rub on each other
and stimulate an inflammation.[113] This would be exquisitely painful
and one wonders how many sufferers permitted it. Other surgeons
threaded a seton (drain) composed of twisted silk threads on a needle
through the cavity between the bone ends to stimulate bone formation. In addition to irritating the bone ends, the exposed drain certainly lead to infection. If the infection was mild and the patient's
resistance and normal defenses overcame the infection, healing might
occur. The introduction of a virulent infection destroyed any chance
of the bone healing and, at best, lead to chronic drainage of pus, and
could even cause septicemia and death of the patient.

Dorsey, in his textbook of surgery, describes a patient treated by
Dr. Physick for a non-union of the humerus who passed a curved needle armed with a twisted silk seton across the non-union and left it in
place.[114] He splinted the arm and dressed it daily. The immediate reaction was drainage of pus, but by twelve to fifteen weeks the bone was
thought to be healed. On April 11, 1801, Isaac Patterson, seaman, aged
twenty-eight, was presented to Physick with a history of a fracture of
his left arm which failed to heal. It had been splinted and a second
reduction had failed to result in healing when Patterson was referred
to Physick. The patient was admitted to Pennsylvania Hospital with
bilious fever and Physick didn't have an opportunity to treat the fracture until December 18, 1802. At that time he passed a needle attached
to a skein of silk through the un-united part of the fracture. As expected, inflammation and pus soon exuded from the needle track and the
wound was dressed and splinted until May 4, 1803, when the wound
closed and the silk was withdrawn.

In 1830 Physick was asked in consultation to see a patient for
remittent fever and he recognized him as the seaman he had operated upon in 1802. The patient reported that in the intervening twenty-
eight years the arm had given him no trouble. Later, the patient died

of the fever and Physick, remembering his training under the cele-brated anatomist John Hunter, got permission to examine the bone. The bone was united with a small hole at the point of union where the silk passed through.[115]

Open fractures were also discussed by Jones in his textbook. Always the teacher, he advised his students:

> "It might also be of singular advantage to young sur-geons, particularly before they begin an operation to go through every part of it attentively in their own minds to consider every possible accident which may happen and to have the proper remedies at hand in case they should; and in all operations of delicacy and difficulty to act with deliberation...."[116]

"When the bone ends are forced through the integument," result-ing in a compound or open fracture, the first consideration is: will the limb survive? Or, it might be added, will the patient survive? Sir Percival Pott taught that the best outcome in this situation was to amputate the limb immediately to prevent general sepsis. Most sur-geons thought this dictum was too radical and made initial efforts to save the limb.

When Pott himself fell and incurred an open fracture of his ankle, he sought out his teacher, Nourse, in London, who suggested nonop-erative management, and his life and limb were saved. This personal experience had little influence, however, on Pott's teaching, and when Bilgauer, the chief military surgeon of the Prussian Army in 1762 directed that a period of observation should precede any amputation for an open fracture, Pott strenuously objected. Baron Van Swieten of Austria also advised waiting and observation for two or three days during which time salt, vinegar and wine were instilled into the wound to protect against putrefaction (infection).[117]

In an earlier period Ambroise Paré also suggested a period of waiting before amputation, if there was no fever. Lastly, the most influential surgeon of that period, John Hunter, also taught delay.

Pott's ideas about amputation for open or compound fractures were influenced by his experiences in crowded London hospitals where nosocomial infections—originating or taking place in a hospital—were rampant. At St. Bartholomew's and St. Thomas', one in every thirteen admissions died. In Paris at the Hotel Dieu, one in five admissions died. In the small country infirmary in England, the death rate was much lower, one in nineteen. The hospital was an incubator, growing a multitude of bacteria from each admission and spreading it to other susceptible patients.

The operation of amputation in itself was a procedure with a high mortality. During the revolution of 1830 in Paris and the riots in 1832, the overall mortality was 39% for major amputations and 52% for thigh amputations. In London the rate was between 45-65%.

Alexander Monro, of the medical school in Edinburgh, provides us with one of the first clinical research projects. In 1737, he did a follow-up study of fourteen consecutive major amputations done at the Edinburgh Royal Infirmary without a hospital mortality. In a later study of ninety-nine major amputations over a fifteen-year span, his mortality in hospital was 8%.[118]

If the surgeon disagreed with Pott and elected to risk the life of the patient to preserve the limb, the factors entering into the decision were the amount of skin and tissue damage, the overall health of the patient, and the area and circumstances of the injury. In open fractures near or through joints and in military operations, amputation was favored. When an attempt was to be made to salvage the limb, fragments of clothing, splinters, soil, and the ball itself, if there was one, were removed from the fracture site, the fracture aligned and reduced visually. If reduction could not be accomplished, the ends of the bone were trimmed to permit such alignment.

After the initial treatment, some surgeons practiced bleeding to offset inflammation, and leeches or a poultice were ordered to reduce the local swelling. To reduce fever, the Peruvian bark (quinine) was given. Fastidious surgeons preserved cleanliness by changing the drainage soiled sheets and the immobilizing pillows frequently.

If amputation was successfully avoided and abscesses developed, they were incised and left open. Chronic drainage or a fistula is irreparable, "for the surgeon is no Creator; he can neither make flesh or bones."[119]

There are some reports of primary or immediate wound closure in a compound fracture in a selected case, the wound being closed with ligatures or tape, but most surgeons did not practice this. Black describes a carpenter who fell three stories and sustained an open fracture of the femur, who was treated with wound closure and splinting, and noted the fracture to unite without complications.[120]

* * * * * *

OBSTETRICS

Throughout recorded history women assisted at childbirth. Women who had many children and were thus experienced in the birth process were sought to assist their younger neighbors. Most often several women responded to a woman in labor. In the fifteenth century, women assisting at delivery were recognized by the Church for their work, which went so far as to sanction them to christen children whose deaths were imminent in the absence of a priest, to save the soul of the child and cheat the devil of his due. It even authorized them to do a Caesarian section on a dead mother if the child was viable.[121] By the eighteenth century some women were recognized for their skill, were frequently called upon, developed a widespread reputation, received payment for their services, and were known as midwives.

In spite of the skills and the eminent reputation of a few, midwives in general had an unsavory reputation, and were looked down upon as ignorant and unskilled, often unable to read, slovenly, and heavy drinkers. They were accused of deserting a woman in labor and lured to another by the promise of higher fees. Their position allowed them to falsify the name of the father and to dispose of unwanted children left in their care. Often they engaged in the trade of selling children to childless couples and some were accused of using their position as procuresses for men. When a child was stillborn or entered the world with unsightly deformities, some members of the community believed they were witches conspiring with the devil. When Ann Hutchinson, in the Massachusetts Bay Colony, challenged the Puritan theocracy, she was accused of witchcraft and expelled from the colony. Margaret Jones, also a midwife, was accused of witchcraft and executed in 1648.

Midwives with a record of delivering sound children and a living mother were those who patiently waited for nature to complete the birth process, confining their activities to comforting and supporting the mother and finally tying the umbilical cord. They knew how long they could delay before calling for help. If the presentation was other than the vertex of the head, they recognized trouble ahead and sent for help immediately. The experienced and conscientious midwife was comfortable with a head presentation, but with a breech or footling presentation, she sensed danger to both the mother and child. The assistance they called was either a more experienced midwife or a physician. The worst midwives were those too impatient to await the natural process, who interfered and who tried various unproven drugs or manipulation. Many tried for many hours to deliver a child without calling for help, knowing they could not give any meaningful help to the mother as precious time passed and the strength of the mother carrying a dead fetus waned.[122]

Early in the eighteenth century books were published in an effort to improve the care rendered by the midwife. An anonymous English physician W:_____ S_____, M.D., claimed to translate the writings of Aristotle on this subject into English. Actually, he cites Hippocrates, his own ideas, and those of his contemporaries, and includes a generous serving of popular folklore. His stated reason for the book is, "It is for your Sakes worthy matrons that I render'd this excellent Treatise in English....". The book is divided into several sections including a review of anatomy of the pelvis and the reproductive organs which would be valuable to those midwives who could read. In other areas it is fanciful, and tells us of local superstitions prevalent in this period.

Conception is described as: "...the parts appointed for generation are a mutual itch which begets in them a Desire for the Action....". Men and women are so driven by the itch, that the consequences are not considered, "but neither sex makes their reflection till after the Action is over....." Successful conception is evidenced if a woman has been very desirous and taken much pleasure in copulation. Conception is further proved if she is cold and chilly afterword and has a loathing for those things she loved before, shows loss of appetite and later becomes nauseated and vomits. Further confirmation is the belly becoming initially flat or engorgement of the veins of the breast, or if the veins under the lower eyelid are swollen. Conception is proven if the urine strained through a linen cloth has small living creatures in it or if a green nettle in the urine kept overnight is full of red spots. Lastly, suppression of the "terms" occurs as the blood is necessary for nourishment of the embryo.

The midwife is also instructed in sex determination. "If it is to be a male the mother's belly is less rounded and higher and the first stirring is on the right while the right nipple is redder. A drop of mother's milk is placed in a basin of water. If it spreads on top, it is a boy, if it sinks it is a girl." This is an infallible sign.[123]

In addition to the section on anatomy, this book does instruct in the lie of the child, the attachments of the placenta, and the risks associated with an unusual presentation, and it discusses some mechanical maneuvers to improve the presenting position of the child. The author disputes Aristotle's ideas of fetal growth by absorbing nutrients through the skin or ingesting them by mouth, and teaches that nourishment reaches the fetus through the "navel vessels" and reveals that he is familiar with the discoveries of Harvey.

A pregnant women was regarded in this century as indisposed and sick for nine months. She must have a good diet, clear air; avoid all ill smells. Even the stink of a partially extinguished candle could cause a miscarriage. Dancing and excessive exercises, and riding in a coach were to be avoided, and she was to abstain from the "...embraces of her husband when with child."

Other texts were published for the instruction of midwives. *The Midwives Companion or a Treatise on Midwifery* was published in 1737. The author in his introduction is euphoric over the marvelous discoveries of this era. "Medicine was at the inception of a new and glorious age, and medical sciences will advance to new heights based on the recent discoveries in the physical sciences." Some ignoramuses may assert, "...that our forefathers were as well skilled in the liberal arts and sciences as the present age." Many physicians in this period expected a quantum leap of medical knowledge equivalent to the physical sciences, but it never was realized.

Again, the author proceeds to flail the midwife, decries the use of any instruments by midwives and blames them for deforming children and killing mothers. "The action of such butcherly midwives ought to be considered murder in plain daylight." On the positive side, he discusses normal birth processes, ovarian tumors and congenital deformities.

This author also reveals to us superstitions widely held in the community. Infertility, like most diseases in this period, was treated by bleeding. The onus of infertility rested with the woman. Some women he says are always barren, some always fertile; though, "I cannot say I ever saw a red haired woman barren, if her husband was anything like a man and within the age of forty five."[124]

Popular belief ascribed deformed children resulting from the mother being frightened or psychologically traumatized. Bracken supported this myth and describes deformity in the newborn as the result of the mother being frightened; the part deformed is the part being formed at the time of the fright. Fear of delivering a deformed child due to events witnessed by the mother prevailed throughout Europe. Louis XIV in France decreed that deformed or lame beggars and freaks were not to be publicly displayed in fairs; and that such people were to be kept in public institutions, out of sight of the populace. Providing care for these people would be praiseworthy if it were humane, but it probably was not.

Congenital lues venera or syphilis was rarely discussed in medical texts of this period where it was thought to be easily overcome by calomel (mercury) pills. Bracken's book describes lues venera as a distemper which any modest woman may receive from a "vicious husband". He correctly recommends that treatment with mercury be started as early as possible in pregnancy to prevent the birth of an infected child.

Another book for instruction of midwives commenced with harsh criticisms of midwives, particularly censoring them for haste, not seeking early assistance, and damning them for the use of instruments which brings the child into the world piecemeal, rather than whole.[125]

In addition to the chastening by the authors of these books and others, woman midwives were challenged by the entry of men into their profession. Men midwives were usually physicians with an obstetrical practice, and a bitter rivalry ensued. Women midwives pointed out that the virtue of mothers was compromised by the male presence; a woman who exposed herself to a male could in the future allow other men similar liberties. The women midwives claimed they brought the womanly traits of compassion and tenderness to the mother and tender, maternal care for the newborn which are attributes alien to men.[126]

Men midwives recounted the long history of grievances held by the public in the past and stated they brought greater knowledge and skill to the mother in labor; moreover they claimed men were more responsible, could more naturally develop a defined course of action, and had knowledge of the use of forceps, in which women were not skilled.

Obstetrical forceps first came on the scene in England and America about 1720. They had been in use for over a hundred years and held as a secret within the Chamberlan family who passed the secret in the family from generation to generation. They were said to have been invented by Peter Chamberlan, a barber-surgeon.[127]

Many arguments centered around the use of obstetrical forceps. Did they solve problems in difficult labor or were they employed to speed up the birth process by an impatient physician, maiming the child and wounding the mother? William Hunter displayed his forceps to his students and proudly pointed out the rust collected on the blades from long periods of disuse. He taught that when they saved one child, they murdered twenty.[128]

The bitter arguments of the men and women midwives reached the membership of the Royal College of Physicians of London. An anonymous author with a sense of satirical humor wrote, "The Petition of the Unborn Babes to the Censors of the Royal College of Physicians", in support of women midwives. The petition declaimed the learning, dexterity and integrity of men midwives and asked them, "to heed the cries of the unborn babes...and yet these men are permitted in their single Opinion avowedly and professedly, to kill our children, to treat our Wives in such a manner as frequently ends in their Destruction, and to have such Intercourse with our Women as easily shifts itself into Indecency, from Indecency into Obscenity and from Obscenity into Debauchery." The accused doctors were Doctors Paulus, Maulus, Barbones, etc.[129]

The unstated reason behind the rivalry was who would collect the fees. Women saw men dispossessing them from a position they had traditionally held since ancient civilization; men feared that women midwives would enlarge their sphere of activities and practice medicine.

With the establishment of lying-in hospitals in Britain at this time, matrons were carefully selected and then given instruction in obstetrics and an opportunity to practice their skills under supervision in a controlled setting. Graduates of these programs diffused throughout the country and raised the standards of practice.

In America, midwives were also subjected to harsh criticism. The male dominated culture of this century taught that the characteristics of a woman disqualified her as a midwife. Women were distinguished for passion and fortitude and sympathy, and because of these emotions, they lacked objectivity.

When a midwife is overcome by complications of labor, physicians claimed, it is too late to call a consultant. The patient's life ebbs before the physician arrives and the facts of the case are communicated to him. Physicians also feared that if women continued to do this work, doctors would lose their skills in this field.[130] The lack of training and skill as well as the indignities to the mother rose to such a pitch in New York that the city felt it necessary to pass an ordinance on July 16, 1716.

> "It is ordained that no woman within this corporation shall exercise the employment of midwife until she has taken oath before the mayor, recorder, or an alderman to the following affect: That she will be diligent and ready to help any woman in labor whether rich or poor; that in time of necessity she will not forsake the poor woman and

go to the rich; that she will not cause or suffer any woman to name or put any father to the child, but only him which is the true father thereof, indeed, according to the utmost of her power; that she will not suffer any woman to pretend to be delivered of a child who is not, indeed, neither to claim any woman's child for her own; that she will not suffer any woman's child to be murdered or hurt; and as often as she shall see one in peril or jeopardy either in the mother or the child, she will call in other midwives for counsel; that she will not administer any medicine to produce a miscarriage; that she will not enforce a woman to give more for her services than is right."[131]

The injustice which the bill seeks to correct signals a widespread lack of ability of the midwives and overcharging their patients; also, the nefarious practice of abandonment of the mother in the middle of labor, fraudulent reporting of the true father, and trumped up deliveries which could lead to child switching or extortion.

William Shippen in Philadelphia gave a series of twenty lectures on midwifery to physicians after his return from Edinburgh. The fame of his lectures, which were illustrated with charts and anatomical drawings, spread throughout the colonies so that his later lectures were attended by as many as 200 students, and drew protests from the community who suspected him of grave robbing to provide material for demonstrations. On several occasions mobs broke into his home and on one occasion he was forced to escape through a back alley.

Shippen had a low opinion of midwives and told his students that he was often called into consultation in cases of difficult labor, "most of which were made so by the unskillful old women...that great suffering of the mother, accompanied by loss of life to them or their offspring have followed, which easily could have been prevented by proper management...."[132]

There are few original records of early American midwives. Elizabeth Coates Paschall (1701-53) probably practiced midwifery, but the eighty pages of her handwritten text is concerned with herbal prescriptions for various illnesses, and it would appear that her practice was more in the field of medicine than midewifery.[133]

Martha Ballard left a diary of her experiences in Augusta, Maine, during the years 1780-1812. She was on call for deliveries and had much experience, but aside from general comments, we are not privileged to learn of her problems and the outcome of her work. She cooperated with the local physicians who regarded her work as satisfactory. Her diary shows that she practiced more medicine than midwifery, treating ailments in children, men and women involving dysentery, and perhaps typhoid fever and scarlet fever, as well as serious local infections. Her obstetrical knowledge was the result of personal experience in giving birth to a large family and her medical practice was based on a self-taught knowledge of herbal medicine. She had no knowledge of anatomy and thus attempted no surgery, nor did she ever employ forceps.[134]

Susanna Müller confined herself to the practice of midwifery in rural Lancaster County, Pennsylvania, during the years 1791-1815. She was more comfortable speaking and writing in German than English and her knowledge of obstetrics was self-taught. She rode horseback on a "swift horse" usually unescorted, at all hours of the day and night, often in extreme weather conditions. In a methodical manner she kept some details of each delivery during the twenty-four years of her service. Her record book shows the date of the delivery, the number of children in the family, the family name and also the fees she received; her charge usually was £7, 6 shillings, although for some unexplained reason she sometimes received £15. On her epitaph it is stated she delivered 1667 children.[135]

* * * * * *

The textbook *Outline of the Theory and Practice of Midwifery* by Alexander Hamilton of the medical staff of Edinburgh was first published in 1775 and was the classic text studied by all students.[136] Even before the publication of his book, he was the recognized authority in this field. In his text he spends much time on disproportion between the size of the fetus and the pelvic dimensions of the mother. The procedures first recommended when there was gross disproportion preventing delivery was division of the symphysis or anterior pelvis to allow it to spread and increase the size of the birth canal.. If the fetus still couldn't pass, he describes embryotomy or the destruction of the embryo so it could be delivered in fragments and allow the mother to survive.

The procedure which he emphatically disapproved was cesarean section, "Where the patient is as it were embowelled alive."[137] Samuel Bard, in America, wrote a textbook on *Midwifery* and noted that some French writers boasted of having performed a caesarian section, but he doubted that a successful procedure, in which both mother and child survived, was ever recorded. "...the event is so generally fatal, if not universally fatal, that the object of the operation is confined to an attempt to save the life of the child after the death of the mother...."[138] It was called, "a detestable barbarous and illegal piece of inhumanity." The only excuse for electing this procedure was when the mother had died or the uterus had ruptured and the child was free in the abdomen.

Hamilton vividly describes a case history where he and his colleagues were forced into a cesarean section: "Elizabeth Clerk, age thirty, having been married several years had a miscarriage in her third month." The expulsion of the fetus severely lacerated her perineum resulting in massive scarring and distortion. She again conceived and

Dr. Hamilton and others were in attendance. "On Monday, 3rd January 1774, about midnight, she was unable to deliver due to her scar and the physicians couldn't even properly examine her, her canal was so distorted. The following day she was brought from the country to the Royal Infirmary in Edinburgh. Upon examination, the pelvis was distorted but the baby was otherwise well-shaped, although a small size." She was operated upon on the 15th of January, 1774.

> "A consultation of surgeons was called and a cesarean section was decided upon. At six in the evening the operator made an incision on the left side of the abdomen in the ordinary way through the integuments...an incision was made into the uterus and a stout male child was extracted from above. The wound was closed by the quill suture and superficially dressed. The patient (without anesthesia) supported the operation with surprising courage and resolution.
>
> Being laid in bed she vomited, complained of chilliness and with application of some heat she slept for four or five hours.
>
> On the 16th about two o'clock she complained of considerable pain on the opposite side for which she was blooded...the pain increased, her pulse became frequent, she was hot and complained of drought. At seven a.m. the injection was repeated but with little success; and at eight more blood was taken from her arm.... She was blooded again at twelve.
>
> At three p.m. her pulse was 136 and she vomited and was given a cordial anodyne, the vomiting abated but the

pulse continued small and the pain and oppressed breathing increased. At seven p.m. her pulse rose to 142 and she called for some bread which she swallowed with difficulty. The drought was intense and she began to toss. Two clysters of warm water with oil were injected without effect. At eight p.m. her belly was tense and swelled as big as before the operation, her pulse was small and feeble; she looked ghastly and expired a little before midnight, twenty-six hours after the operation."[139]

The surgeons at Edinburgh couldn't find any reason why this cesarean section fared so badly. Some suggested it was uterine irritation, internal hemorrhage, or flooding of the abdomen with fluid from the uterus or the usual comment about admitting air into the abdomen.

Numerous experiments were done on animals and it was concluded that after a large abdominal wound which is quickly and accurately closed, the animals generally survived, but if the bowel was exposed for a longer period to the cold air, "dreadful inflammation" occurred.

Elisabeth Clerk almost certainly died of a bacterial peritonitis. The operation was performed technically satisfactorily; a live child was delivered, the placenta totally removed, the wound remained closed, no evisceration is reported, and severe hemorrhage did not occur. The little "animals" seen drifting about under Van Leeuwenhoek's microscope were regarded as fascinating to watch, but no one appreciated that they could cause the "dreadful inflammation" that killed Elisabeth Clerk.

In America, as in Britain, Hamilton's *Outline of Midwifery* was the standard text. In 1790 it was printed in Philadelphia and widely distributed, and its strong denunciation of cesarean section was common teaching. After the war, Samuel Bard published his text, which reaffirmed Hamilton's conclusions.

370 *Medical Observations and Inquiries.*

was more diſordered in this, than in her former pregnancy, frequently feveriſh, the ſwelling of her belly not ſo equal, nor the motion of the child ſo ſtrong and lively. At the end of nine months, when ſhe expected her delivery, ſhe had ſome labour-pains, but without a flow of waters, or any other diſcharge. The pains ſoon went off, and the ſwelling of her belly grew gradually leſs ; but there ſtill remained a large, hard, indolent, moveable tumour, inclining a little to the right ſide. She had a return of her *menſes*, continued regular five months, conceived again, and enjoyed better health: the ſwelling of her belly became more equal and uniform, and, at the end of nine months, after a ſhort and eaſy labour, ſhe was delivered of a healthy child. The tumour on the right ſide had again the ſame appearances as before her laſt pregnancy. Five days after delivery, ſhe was ſeized with a violent fever, a purging, ſuppreſſion of the *lochia*, pain in the tumour, and profuſe fetid ſweats. By careful treatment, theſe threatening ſymptoms were, in ſome meaſure, removed ; but there ſtill remained

Medical Obſervations and Inquiries. 369

XXXII. *A caſe of an extra-uterine fœtus, deſcribed by Mr. John Bard, Surgeon at New York ; in a letter to Dr. John Fothergill, and by him communicated to the Society.*

Read March 24, 1760.

SIR,

DR. Colding, ſome time ago, ſhewed me a letter he was favoured with from you ; wherein you acquaint him with the deſign of publiſhing the London Medical Eſſays ; and invite him to encourage that work, by communicating any uſeful or curious obſervations, which might fall under his notice in this part of the world. Encouraged by this invitation to the Doctor, whom I have the honour to be intimate with, I have taken the freedom, though a ſtranger, to ſend you the hiſtory of a caſe, which has lately fallen under my care.

Mrs. STAGG, the wife of a maſon, about 28 years of age, having had one child without any uncommon ſymptom, either during her pregnancy or labour, became, as ſhe imagined, a ſecond time pregnant. She was

VOL. II.   Bb

An four-page article by John Bard M.D. of New York in which he described the first operation for removal of an extra-utering pregnancy; published in Dr. John Fothergill's Observations in London. (continued on opposite page.)

Jessee Bennett graduated from the University of Pennsylvania where Hamilton's *Outline of Midwifery* was used, and then established his practice in 1794 in a remote area of western Virginia in the Shenandoah Valley, caring for his young wife now at term. Her contracted pelvis prevented normal delivery and he watched frantically

Medical Observations and Inquiries, 271

a loss of appetite, flow hectic fever, night sweats, and a *diarrhœa*. To the tumour, which continued painful, and gradually increased, were applied fomentations, and emollient pultices; and, at the end of nine weeks, I perceived so evident a fluctuation of matter in it, that I desired Dr. Huck, physician to the army, to visit this patient with me, and be present at the opening it. From the whole history we concluded, that we should find an extra-uterine *fœtus*. I made an opening in the most prominent part of the tumour, about the middle of the right *rectus* muscle, beginning as high as the navel, and carrying it downwards. There issued a vast quantity of extremely fetid matter, together with the third *phalanx* of a finger of a child. Introducing my finger into the abscess, I found an opening into the cavity of the *abdomen* by the side of the *rectus* muscle, through which I felt the child's elbow. I then directed my incision obliquely downwards to the right *ilium*, and extracted a *fœtus* of the common size, at the ordinary time of delivery. The frontal, parietal, and occipital bones, as also

the

B b 2

372 *Medical Observations and Inquiries.*

the third *phalanges* of the fingers of one hand, separated by putrefaction, remained behind; which I also took out. We imagined the *placenta* and *funis umbilicalis* were dissolved into *pus*, of which there was a great quantity. By the use of fomentations and detersive injections, while the discharge was copious, fetid, and offensive; and by the application of proper bandages, and dressing with dry lint only, when the *pus* became laudable, the cavity contracted, filled up, and was cicatrized in ten weeks. The force of the hectic being removed, with the help of the bark, *elix.* of *vitriol*, and a proper diet, she quickly recovered good health. Her milk, which had left her from the time she was first seized with the fever, returned in great plenty after the abscess was healed; and she now suckles a healthy infant.

New York,
Dec. 25, 1759.

I am,
S I R,
With great respect,
Your most humble servant,
JOHN BARD.

for several days as his wife weakened. Bennett was distraught and consulted with another physician, Dr. Humphreys, in a neighboring community. A cesarean section seemed to be the only solution in spite of the dire warnings in the textbooks. He placed a crude plank atop two barrels in his log cabin and helped his exhausted wife to lie on the plank. Opium was given in place of an anesthetic. Assisted by his sister and a black servant, he laid open the abdomen and uterus with one stroke of the blade and delivered his daughter. Before closing the wound he "spayed" his wife, remarking that if she lived, neither of them could bear such an ordeal the second time. The mother survived and the daughter lived to the age of seventy-seven years.[140]

Bennett never reported this operation and it came to light much later in the nineteenth century from reports of his sister and other doctors in the community. When asked why he never reported the operation, Bennett replied, "no doctor with any feeling of delicacy would report an operation on his wife." He did write, "the operation is not essentially mortal."[141]

Elsewhere in Virginia, William Baynham practiced obstetrics and was known throughout the South. Baynham had studied with John Hunter at St. Thomas in London and was made an assistant professor of anatomy in Cambridge where he remained for sixteen years and received his membership as a Fellow of the Royal College before deciding to return home. On two occasions in Virginia he successfully operated upon women with ectopic pregnancies; the cases were reported in the Philadelphia Journal of Medical and Physical Sciences.[142]

Earlier in New York, John Bard was asked to see a young woman with a mass in her abdomen, noted nine months after she delivered her second normal child. Bard was so convinced that she carried an extrauterine dead fetus that he operated on her. Upon entering the abdomen, he found a dead, macerated fetus, which he successfully removed. A report of this unusual operation was published in Fothergill's *Medical Observations and Inquiries* on March 24, 1760.[143, 144]

Postchildbirth infection, puerperal sepsis, was the feared complication of childbirth. Long before knowledge of the bacterial cause of this condition, Ignaz Semmelweis in Vienna in the mid nineteenth century described how it reaped its greatest toll in large city hospitals and that it was spread by physicians failing to wash their hands between examinations. Many years before, in 1798, Hubard, in Philadelphia, also described its high incidence in crowded cities and that it rarely occurred in the country. Hubard, who was singularly perceptive and beyond his time, wrote, "I am however, inclined to believe that it has been...the effect of a peculiar contagion or infection than of any change produced in the air."[145]

CHAPTER THREE

POPULAR MEDICINE

Nature Does Nothing Rashly
Too Much of Anything is an Enemy of Nature.
John Archer

Common sense was the second rule of health; the first was to be God-fearing. "When man came first out of the hands of the Creator, clothed in body as well as in soul with immortality and incorruption, there was no place for physick...or the art of healing. As he knew no sin, so he knew no sickness, weakness or body disorder. There was no decay in his environment and nothing without to injure him. The entire creation was at peace with man as long as man was at peace with his Creator. When man rebelled against the Sovereign of heaven and earth, immortality was lost and sickness and death must be expected."[146] The author of these words singled out the Americans as those who were best able to survive under these circumstances because of their vigorous life. "The Americans have few diseases because of their continual exercises and temperance."

Most people couldn't afford doctor's fees, and moreover they had little faith in the physician's ability to cure disease, preferring instead to trust the many healers who advertised their remedies and printed books on self-care. Some doctors gained notoriety and their books were much in demand. John Colbatch, in his book, *Medicine Made Easy*, told the public, "The Science of Physic is not so great a Mystery (although industriously clouded by the Sons of the Art), but anyone may with little Pains and Attention fall in with the most proper method to Preserve Health or restore it in a case of Sickness."[147] According to the author the cause of all disease is the entrance into the blood or juices of some gross matter, so coarse it lodges in the vessels and other organs and health is not restored until the offending material is evacuated.

Wesley's book on self-medication in 1772 was reprinted fifteen times and strongly emphasized a simple, sparing lifestyle with fresh air, exercise, and cleanliness. The book offers prescriptions for each illness: "For an ague take a cold bath and then handful of yarrow and onion, cover with a thin linen and place the whole in a paper bag with holes and wear it on the pit of the stomach, replacing it every two hours." "To prevent rickets in children dip them in cold water every morning until age eight or nine." For the bite of a mad dog, "a pound of salt and a quart of water squeezed into the wound for one hour, then bind salt on the wound. N.B. The Author of this recipe was bit six times by mad dogs and always cured."[148]

Most Americans living on farms in remote communities didn't have easy access to a doctor, nor could they afford the fees demanded for professional services. Within each household some member was concerned with illness and cures; most likely the family matriarch, who carefully read the medical anecdotes of the farmer's almanac. She traded her knowledge of cures with others in the area and could assign certain symptoms to be offset by medications. Some person in the village had a copy of a medical text written for the use of the laity and could compare the symptoms of the patient with a prescription set forth to relieve these symptoms. Making a diagnosis was irrelevant except in cases of smallpox, measles and a few other commonly encountered and easily recognized diseases. The village minister or shoemaker or some other trusted person who had a reputation for cures would be consulted, and the sick neighbor placed full confidence in his nostrums. The season of the year, the state of the weather, and the signs of the zodiac played a role in the selection of proper treatment. When the patient failed to respond, outside help would be sought. Such a person could be an untrained, self-styled doctor, often selling a secret remedy, or it could be an apprentice who received his training from another doctor with whom he studied for up to seven years. Lastly, the doctor could be a graduate of a medical school either in America or abroad. There were few well-trained physicians in rural America; most plied their trade in the cities along the seaboard.

One of the more scientific books available to rural Americans was the *American Domestick Medicine*, which was designed for family use and included chapters on basic anatomy, fortuitous diseases (consumption, pleurisy, colic, etc.) and habitual diseases (recurrent). There were also chapters on childhood diseases, women's diseases, pregnancy and parturition. Each specific condition had its own prescription.[149]

A prescription could be lengthy and complicated. For example:

> "For an ague and to restore limbs and loins lamed through the gout; take a foxe and draw out the entrailes, then take Sage, Rosemary, Juniper leaves and berries, Dill, wilde marjoram of the garden, Lavender, Chamomile of each halfe a pound, Stampe these herbes in a mortar of stone very finely, then cut the foxe in pieces and put him with the herbes in a vessel of eight gallons and put to foure pints of Oyle of olive, Oyle of Neate's feet, calves suet, Deer suet, Goose grease, Brocke's grease

of each one pound, and a halfe of sea water three quartes and as much as good malmsey, set all together on the fire and baile it till the wine and water be consumed and that the flesh and bones be separated asunder; then take it from the fire and straine it and presse it through strong canvasse cloth and so reserve it to your use as an oynt-ment against all aches."[150]

Another widely used book of receipts (recipes) by Moncrief[151] has an appendix of secret prescriptions by Archibald Pitcairn, "that great ornament of his Country and incomparable physician." Another popular book, *Rational Physic and a Family Dispensatory*, was expressly written for people too distant from the services of a physician or who couldn't afford a physician.[152] Written in simple non-technical language it doesn't discuss causes of diseases and confines itself to treatment of symptoms, but it teaches how to take the pulse, and the significance of a quick, slow, full, or weak pulse. The reader is instructed how to look at the tongue (red, inflamed, swollen), the urine (bloody, coffee ground, yellow or brown), and the stool (looseness, bloody, odorous). After doing your own examination, you consult the various symptoms and signs for the proper prescription.

A prescription for lovesickness:

"Hereos is the Greke worde —
In Latin it is named amor
In English it is named "Love Sicke"
    and women may have this fickness as well as men
Young perfons be much troubled with this impediment

The Caufe Of This Infirmitie
The infirmitie doth come of amours which is a fervant love for to have carnal copulation with the party that is

loved: and it cannot be obteyned -

fome be so foolifh that they be ravifhed of their wyttes

A REMEDY

First I do advertife every perfon not to fet to the hart

that another fet to the hele -

Let no man fet his hart fo far but that he may withdraw

it betime, and mufe not;

But ufe mirth and merry company and be wife and not

foolifh

ANOTHER REMEDY - SATYRIAFIS

Leap into a great veffel of cold water and applying

nettles to the offending part[153]

From a medical text by Andrew Bode - 1549

Quote by John Aiken in *Memoirs of Medicine -"*

These manuals taught the "manner and way of compounding all such oyles, unguents, sirrups, cataplasms, waters, powders, emplasters, pills and etc. as shall be useful in any private house with little labour, small cash, and in short time." Some books offer advice on regaining strength and discuss sleep, diet, rest, work, proper air, and exercise as well as moderation in venery: "But that sleep in the night time be counted and esteemed wholesome; yet except if it be restrained within certaine limits, it will prove otherwise. Therefore eight houres is sufficient, for longer times, hinders the evacuation." Discussing too much sex, "The immoderate use of venery produces divers discomodities as the faintness of the spirits, forgetfulness, loss of sight,....cramps, running of the reines, pissing of blood, shedding urine involuntary, and divers times, the French pox with ulceration of the privities."[154] A prescription for this condition employs juice of plantain, sheep's milk, bone of armoniack, decoctions of knob grass, horse tail, purslaine and bramble tops. Later the pox was treated with prescriptions including mercury. "To multiply the hair, apply burnt ashes of goat's dung anointed with oil and applied to scalp."

In addition to lengthy prescriptions, phlebotomy or blood letting and cupping were recommended for some symptoms such as a heavy pulse. A head vein should be opened for a headache, the left arm for lung disease, the right arm for the liver, for gait disturbances the veins of the part afflicted.

Phlebotomy was first "invented by the river horse of the Nile (hippopotamus) who relieved excess blood and humors by rubbing the thigh against a rough section of the river bank, and after bleeding sufficiently, stops the bleeding by rolling in the mud."[155]

Boxing or cupping is for evacuation of toxic humors. The recommended method is to put a little wax into a glass, light the wax, and apply firmly to the skin of the ailing part. After the glass falls off, scarify the skin with a knife and reapply the glass with a lighted wax so blood with humors is withdrawn. Leeches can substitute for cupping, but only certain kinds of leeches are usable and they must be applied carefully without the leech touching the skin of the treater or it refuses to collect blood from the patient.[156]

A widely used medical textbook in Britain and America was written in 1742 by Thomas Dover; in one volume it contains a compendium of all the diseases of mankind. The preface says the book describes, "Diseases incident to mankind, described in so plain a manner that any Person may know the nature of his own Disease." Testimonials are used to increase the confidence of the reader. For example: "Yet Mr. Towne, one of the kings gardeners, died of it (dropsy) under Dr. Radcliffe's care." The patient was initially seen by Dr. Dover but refused to accept his advice. The first part of the book discusses dropsy, diabetes, consumption, asthma, hypochondriasis in men and hysteria in women; there are chapters on gout and the king's evil (scrofula). The second part of the book lists prescriptions for each of these conditions.[157]

The Ancient

PHYSICIAN's

Legacy to his Country.

Being what he has collected himself,

In Fifty-eight Years PRACTICE:

Or, an Account of the several

DISEASES incident to Mankind;

Described in so plain a Manner,

That any Person may know the Nature of his own Disease.

Together with the several Remedies for each Distemper, faithfully set down.

Designed for the Use of all Private Families.

Homines ad Deos, nullâ in re propius accedunt, quam Salutem hominibus dando. Cic.

Homines ad Dæmona, nullâ in re propius accedunt, quam Salutem hominibus negando. Do.

By THOMAS DOVER, M. B.

The Sixth Edition.

In this Edition are very considerable Additions; besides a great Number of Letters sent from several Parts of *England*, of the extraordinary Cures perform'd by Crude Mercury: With some Remarks on the Author of *The Use and Abuse of Mercury.* To which is added, An Essay on *Midwifry*; and the *Moral Converfation* of the College of Physicians, in *Latin* and *English*, by Way of Appendix; together with a *Digreffion.*

LONDON:
Printed by H. Kent, for C. Hitch at the *Red-Lyon* in *Pater-Nofter-Row*; J. Brotherton at the *Bible*, next the *Fleece* Tavern in *Cornhill*; and R. Minors, in St. *Clement's* Church-Yard, in the *Strand.* M.DCC.XLII.

Price ftitch'd, Four Shillings,

Title page of a popular book for self treatment published in the 1740s.

Poor Richard's Almanacks, sold in Philadelphia by Benjamin Franklin, published articles on treatment for many maladies. In the *Pennsylvania Gazette* of December 16 to December 23, 1736, an advertisement requests the reader to purchase the *Almanack* to learn how to deal with snakebites. "Just Published *Poor Richard's Almanack* for the year 1737, containing besides what is useful, a particular description of the Herb which the Indians used to cure the bites of the venomous Reptile a Rattlesnake, an exact print of the leaf of the plant, an Account of the places it grows in and the manner of using it...."

In the February 12th issue of 1774 one read, *"Poor Richard's Almanack* containing besides the usual astronomical observations, Dr. Tissot's remarks on Persons Drowned, and some rules of Practice for the recovery of such unhappy sufferers.... Receipts to clean the Teeth and Gums and make the flesh grow close to the enamel—a sure preservative against the toothache.... Remedy of corns,...for the rheumatism and the ague.... Cure for the yellow jaundice. And excellent receipt for the cure of consumption...for a sorethroat...for the cure of worms in horses."

In the July 13, 1774, issue, "Dr. Geo Weed begs leave to inform the public that the following medicines have had so great a success in resolving of those disorders they are prescribed for, that people are continually applying for them, which gives him great satisfaction to think he was made an instrument under God to administer any relief to those who were under painful disorders.

"Syrup and Powder to cure the bloody flux.

"Royal Balsam cures all kinds of wounds and bruises and helps back pain and weakness, cures corns, pleuritic disorders, mortification...."[158]

Apothecaries in Europe and America eagerly sought Indian herbal medicines for use in the treatment of many diseases. Medical practice in Europe and America was dependent on herbs and plants, and the

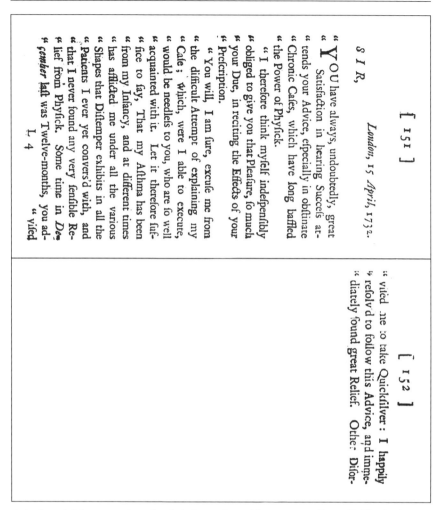

[151]

London, 15 April, 1732.

S I R,

" YOU have always, undoubtedly, great
" Satisfaction in hearing Succeſs at-
" tends your Advice, eſpecially in obſtinate
" Chronic Caſes, which have long baffled
" the Power of Phyſick.
" I therefore think myſelf indeſpenſibly
" obliged to give you that Pleaſure, ſo much
" your Due, in reciting the Effects of your
" Preſcription.
" You will, I am ſure, excuſe me from
" the difficult Attempt of explaining my
" Caſe; Which, were I able to execute,
" would be needleſs to you, who are ſo well
" acquainted with it. Let it therefore ſuf-
" fice to ſay, That my Aſthma has been
" from my Infancy, and at different times
" has afflicted me under all the various
" Shapes that Diſtemper exhibits in all the
" Patients I ever yet convers'd with, and
" that I never found any very ſenſible Re-
" lief from Phyſick. Some time in De-
" cember laſt was Twelve-months, you ad-
L. 4   " viſed

[152]

" viſed me to take Quickſilver : I happily
" reſolv'd to follow this Advice, and imme-
" diately found great Relief. Othe: Diſor-

A testimonial from a patient slowly being poisoned by mercury. *Dover T. The Ancient Physicians Legacy to his Country.* Chas Kent London 1742.

discovery of a new continent, with its previously unknown plants and an indigenous population which was using them, precipitated an intensive search for new cures. Tobacco, sassafras and American ginseng were used as tonics, and shiploads of these plants were exported to Europe, and in the case of ginseng to the Orient, where it was used for respiratory ailments. Sassafras was prescribed for infections, rheumatism, and against moths and bedbugs; maidenhair fern was used as an hemostatic or to check bleeding. John Bartram was encouraged by the Royal Geographic Society to explore the plant life of America and sent boxes to London each containing 100 seeds gathered in his travels in the eastern coastal areas of North America for a guinea each, from where they were distributed throughout Europe. His seed packets were so valued that he was appointed botanist and naturalist to the king, receiving an honorarium of £50 a year.[159]

There was no dearth of a sure cure for any disease. Cures were promised in newspaper advertisements or pamphlets. Thomas Anderton, a glazier turned physician, advertised his services in the *Pennsylvania Gazette*. Specializing in venereal diseases, he sold medications "...that will effectually and radically cure every symptom of the venereal disease without pain or sickness or any confinement. Salivation is wholly by them rendered unnecessary, and they undoubtedly will cure when that fails. They are taken by the most delicate of both sexes at all seasons of the year...; for they improve and invigorate the nervous system."[160] Mercury was the most common drug prescribed for syphilis and salivation was an unpleasant complication of this treatment.

Pamphlets circulated throughout the colonies recommending patent medicines, secret cures and how to prevent disease. *Maxims on the Preservation of Health and the Prevention of Disease* captured the interest and enticed the reader with several pages of quotations by Dr. Franklin before it launched into its sales pitch. "Hamilton's Worm Destroying Lozenges" will cure anyone of worms." It describes an innkeeper suffering from tapeworms. After the first lozenge, four yards of a tapeworm were removed, but the residual "monstrous reptile returned, tearing and clawing his bowels," until another lozenge removed the remaining six to eight yards. "Hamilton's Essence and Extract of Mustard" was advertised as a safe and effective remedy for rheumatism, gout, palsy, lumbago, numbness, white swellings, chilblains, sprains, bruises, pain in the face and neck, and could be administered both internally and externally.

Finally, "Dr. Hamilton's Grand Restorative" was sold for relief and cure of various complaints resulting from "dissipated pleasure, juvenile indiscretions, intoxication, or destructive intemperance, the diseases peculiar to females, lying's in, etc."[161]

Quacks or self-styled healers were increasing at such an alarming rate in the eighteenth century and extorting such large amounts of money from an irate public that critical articles were published against them in newspapers. In the *Boston Weekly Letter* of December 19-January 5, 1737, there was an article asking for legislation that "would exterminate the shoemakers, weavers and almanack makers who were practicing medicine." It recommended that quacks whose treatment resulted in manslaughter ought to be sent to the gallows after two offenses.

The article pointed out that, in the mother country, the Royal College of Physicians in London was empowered by Parliament to approve of anyone practicing medicine for a radius of seven miles around the city and the offender would suffer a fine of 100 shillings for each month of illegal practice. The college later certified physicians throughout England. The newspaper requested such a law in Massachusetts. A previous Massachusetts law passed in 1649 offered some protection to the patient but did not require certification of healers.

In November, 1781, the legislature approved the incorporation of the Massachusetts Medical Society and further stated, "Be it therefore enacted by the Authority foresaid, that the President and Fellows of such society or others such as their officers as they shall appoint have full Power and Authority to examine all Candidates for the practice of Physic and Surgery (who shall offer themselves for Examination in respecting their skill in their Profession) and if upon such Examination the said candidate shall be found skilled in their

Profession and fitted for the Practice of it, they shall receive the Approbation of the Society in Letter Testimonial of such an Examination and the Seal of the Society."[162]

Healers continued to treat much of the American population, gradually losing credibility, but faith healers, patent medicines, and secret remedies persisted well into the twentieth century. Books on health care, particularly on diet and exercise, continue to occupy the shelves of booksellers. Most of these are firmly based on accepted medical information, but some rely on anecdotal experience and unproven theories. A fertile field for such books continues in those areas where modern medicine has failed to successfully treat disease.

CHAPTER FOUR

MEDICAL EDUCATION
IN THE COLONIAL PERIOD

"He, that sinneth before his Maker, let him fall into the hands of a physician. Frequently, there is more danger from the physician than the distemper." Dr. William Douglass, a graduate of Leyden and Paris, had this to say after his settling in Boston in 1718. Douglass was appalled by the large number of physicians without training, preying upon the public. Douglas continued, "In general, the practice of physic in our colonies is so perniciously bad, that excepting in surgery and some acute (surgical cases), it is better to let nature take her own course than to trust the honesty and sagacity of the practitioner."[163] Douglass was arrogant and argumentative and didn't get along even with the best-educated physicians in Boston, one of whom was Zabdiel Boylston, who advocated smallpox inoculation and was viciously attacked by Douglass.

It was said of Douglass: he was always positive, sometimes accurate. Douglass surely overstated his case, but throughout the colonies anyone could call himself a physician, treat patients and dearly sell his secret remedies.

Note that Douglas excluded surgeons from his charge of incompetence. The diagnosis and treatment of a musket or arrow wound, or a fracture, or leg ulcer is usually self-evident and not based on a holistic philosophy or a theory of disease, such as was practiced by most physicians in this period. Most medical treatment was rationalization; surgical treatment was empirical.

Soon after the colonies were established, medical treatment was given by the clergy who were well educated and had a smattering of materia medica, natural history and biology. The medical and religious functions of the clergy often competed for their attention. A theological physician giving his Sunday sermon had a message delivered to the pulpit, stating a girl was seriously ill, and needed his attention promptly. Unable to leave the church, he hastily scribbled a note on the flyleaf of his hymn book, "Let the wench be blooded and wait until I come," passed the note to the messenger and continued his sermon.[164] Other educated people also served as physicians when requested. Governor Edward Winslow of Plymouth included the Indian Chief Massasoit as his patient and the colony remained on good terms with this tribe for many years.[165]

Diseases of Indians and Indian customs attracted the attention of John Josselyn, who made voyages to America in 1638 and 1663. Following the settlement at Plymouth, the colonists shared their disease problems with the Indians. In 1638 Josselyn writes, "The Indians at the Massachusetts were at that time by sickness decreased from 30,000 to 300." The susceptible population readily succumbed to smallpox and "plague". Josselyn also described Indians with consumption, pestilent fever, falling sickness (epilepsy) and the king's evil (scrofula or tuberculosis, which in Europe supposedly could be cured by the touch of a king).

Indian physicians were priests called "powaws" and treated

their patients with charms and herbal medicine. Indians suffering from the plague or smallpox covered their wigwam with strips of bark to prevent any circulation of the air and made a great fire inside until they were in a sweat, then ran down to the sea or a river for a plunge and returned to their wigwam to recover, or give up the ghost.

If they consulted the powaws, Josselyn describes the treatment: "...they place the sick upon the ground sitting, and dance in an antick manner around about him beating their naked breasts and making hideous faces." If recovery occurred, the patient deposited rich gifts of bows and arrows, wampum and beaver skins into a deep hole in a vast rock into which payment was thrown.

"Wives, they have two or three." When their time comes, they would go alone to a suitable bush or tree, lay down and were delivered in "...a trice not so much as groaning for it." Older people living beyond their time and becoming a burden would be starved to death or buried alive. The dead were buried in a deep hole on their "breeches" in a fetal position.

Syphilis was first recognized in Europe in the sixteenth century and a lively debate of whether it originated in Europe or America is frequently encountered in the literature of the period. Josselyn discussed the question of where in Europe syphilis was first seen. He joined those who claim it originated from the American Indians. "The great pox (syphilis) is proper to them by reason...which disease was brought amongst our Europeans, first by the Spanish of that went with Christopher Columbus who brought it to Naples with the Indian women of Italians and French conversed, Ann Dom, 1493, but all agree that it was not known in Europe before Columbus his voyage to America."[166]

* * * * * *

Early medical instruction in Massachusetts can be traced back to 1629 soon after the Plymouth Bay Colony was founded. The director of the New England Company was concerned not only about providing medical care to the colonists and Indians, but also with the training of future doctors. In a letter written in 1647, he wrote, "We have entertained Lambert Wilson, chirurgeon, to remain with yu in the service of the plantation with whom wee are agreed that hee shall serve this Companie and the other planters that li(ve) in the plantation for 3 years and in that tyme apply himself to cure, but also for the indians as from tyme to tyme, and moreover he is to educate and instruct in this Art one or more youths—."[167]

Eighteen years later Giles Firmin had completed a course in anatomy to students in the colony. In a letter to the Minister of Cambridge, dated September 24, 1647, the Apostle Eliot wrote, "Our young students in physick may be trained up better than yet they bee, who have only theoreticall knowledge and are force to fall to practise before they ever saw an Anatomy made or duely trained up in making experiments, for we never had but one Anatomy in the Countrey which Mr. Giles Firmin (now in England) did make and read upon very well, but no more of that now." To Firmin must be accorded the honor of conducting the first medical lectures in America.

Several weeks later on October 26, 1647, the General Court of Massachusetts approved such study of physick and agreed to, "...anatomize once in foure yeares some malefactor[168] in cases these be such in the courte shall allow of."

* * * * * *

Medical treatment for the colonists in addition to that provided by the Plymouth Bay Company was also provided by the Dutch East India Company, which sent contract physicians to their colonies who remained for brief periods. The colonists themselves were forced to look after their own illnesses and misfortunes in the absence of physicians and often performed emergency surgery to the best of their ability.

When Penelope Stout set out to pick beach plums on Sandy Hook Island, and was attacked by a band of Indians who slashed her abdomen and left her for dead with her viscera protruding, she was found by two hunters. They revived her, repacked her viscera into her abdomen, and closed the wound with strips of clothing. She was then transported to the nearest village. The closure was successful and she lived to the age of ninety-four and had four children.[169]

The first operation in the colonies may have been done by Dr. Griffith Owens in 1699. Owens came to America with William Penn, who was being honored on the occasion of his landing in Chester, Pennsylvania. The incident is related by Thomas Story, a witness to the event. "The next day being the first of the tenth month (Dec. 1699, old style) we went over Chester Creek in a boat to the town, and as the Governor landed (William Penn's second visit), some young men, officiously and contrary to express command of some of the magistrates, fired two small sea pieces of cannon and being ambitious of making three out of two, by firing one twice, one of the young men darting in a cartridge of powder, before the piece was sponged had his arm shot to pieces upon which a surgeon being sent for on the ship, then riding, an amputation of the member was quickly resolved on by Dr. Griffith Owens, the surgeon, and some other skilful persons present. But as the arm was cut off, some spirits in a basin happened to catch fire and being spilt on the surgeon's apron set his clothes on fire, and there being a great crowd of spectators, some of them were in the way and in danger of being scalded, as was the surgeon himself was upon the face and hands, but running into the street, the fire was quenched and so quick was he that the patient lost not very much blood though left in that open bleeding condition."[170]

In the early Colonial period anyone so inclined could practice medicine. As quackery reigned with nostrums and secret remedies became widespread, the public increasingly complained of the treatment and the costs. The opinion of the people regarding the efficacy of treatment and the healers code of behavior is well expressed by a writer, who scourged the profession in a letter to the *Charleston Gazette*. "I shall only observe that it has been a Question Whether Lawyers or Physicians did the greatest mischief to men; one impairs their Estates, the other their Health and Life, and then I have somewhere read of a man who fancied himself sick and sent for his physician who asked the patient if he ate well?—He answered yes: Do you drink well?—Yes. Do you sleep well? He still answered—yes. Very well, said the doctor, I'll send you something to remove these disorders!!"[171]

The Virginia Commonwealth, reacting to a complaining public, passed an act on October 21, 1639, to "Compel Physicians and Surgeons to Disclose on Oath the Value of their Medicines." A second act was passed in 1736 by the Virginia Commonwealth, regulating fees and accounts of Physicians—a fee schedule. Each visit and prescription in town was to be five shillings. For every mile of travel one shilling was to be added. Treatment of a simple fracture was to cost two pounds, a compound fracture four pounds. For those with a degree from a university, every visit was ten shillings.

Other restrictive laws regulating the practice of medicine were also recorded. A law was passed by the Massachusetts Bay Colony in 1649 stating, "It is therefore ordered that no person or persons whatsoever employed at any time about the bodies of man, woman or child for preservation of life and health as chirurgeons, midwives, physicians or others, presume to exercise or put forth any act contrary to the known or approved rules of the art in each mystery or occupation, nor exercise any force, violence or cruelty upon or towards the body...." This was the era of the witchhunt. The approved rules of the art would exclude the practice of supernatural powers. New York also faced the problem of errant physicians.[172]

"Few physicians among us are eminent for their skill. Quacks abound like locusts in Egypt. The Profession is under no kind of regulation. We have no laws protecting the King's subjects from the malpractice of the pretender. Any man sets up as physician, surgeon, apothecary. No candidates are either examined or licensed."[173] William Livingstone wrote thus about the quacks and healers in New York in the *Independent Reflector* in 1753. "No man is of greater service or detriment to society than a Physician. If he is skillful, industrious and honest he is of unshakable Benefit to Mankind, but if incapacity, idleness and Roguery are his characteristics, he is a curse to the community...there is no city in the world, not larger than ours, that abounds with so many doctors...the greatest part of them are mere Pretenders to a Profession of which they are entirely ignorant."

Following this article and others, New York passed the first law in the colonies regulating medical practitioners by requiring an examination to obtain a license to practice medicine in 1760.

> "No person whatsoever shall practice as a physician and surgeon in the City of New York before he shall be examined in physics and surgery and approved of and admitted by one of his majesty's council, the judges of the supreme court, the King's attorney general and the mayor of the City of New York for the time being or by any three or more of them taking to their assistance for such examination such proper person or persons as they in their discretion shall think fit."[174]

In 1772 a similar law was passed in New Jersey and later in Massachusetts. After the battles of Concord and Lexington, thousands of militiamen besieged Boston. Filth followed by disease claimed many lives and eroded the army. The Provincial Congress of Massachusetts passed a law on May 8, 1775, whereby medical applicants for the post of regimental surgeons in the militia must pass an examination. James Thacher, having completed his apprenticeship in January 1775 at the age of twenty-one, applied for military service soon after hostilities began in the spring of 1775. He was one of sixteen candidates, and describes his tensions and the nervousness of the group awaiting the examination committee. The examination was to include subjects in anatomy, physiology, surgery and medicine. Six of the sixteen were disqualified and Thacher describes his elation on his successful appointment to the Cambridge hospital under the direction of Dr. John Warren.[175]

Most doctors in America were trained as apprentices. They applied to an established practitioner who might have one or more additional apprentices between the ages of fourteen and seventeen and remained for several years, often as many as five. When accepted, they signed an indenture which stated that they must dedicate themselves to the exclusive task of serving their master. The agreement insisted they behave in an exemplary manner, reveal none of the master's secrets, do his bidding, avoid marriage, do no gambling, and conserve the master's property. At the expiration of his term of indenture, he received a sum of money, usually one hundred pounds, and a certificate stating he had satisfactorily completed his service.

During the early years of his service he would clean the office, saddle and care for his master's horse, and even assist the mistress in household duties. He was provided with books to study in his spare time. Later he would compound medicines and accompany the doctor on his visits and assist in office practice.[176] Most physicians accepted the responsibility to train their apprentices in good faith, while others took gross advantage of their apprentices. John Bard was bound as an apprentice at the age of fourteen to Dr. Kearsley in Philadelphia, who forced him to do the most menial tasks. He had time to study only after the Kearsley family went to bed and considered breaking his contract and leaving many times, but for his mother, who was widowed and supporting three children.[177]

Apprentices were acquainted with anatomy, had reading knowledge of materia medica, and knew of Harvey's discovery of circulation, but rarely did they have practical experience in dissection or the advantage of classroom lectures. They emulated the theories and practice of their preceptors, were cautious and conscientious, and developed a strong bond with their patients. After receiving his certificate, the apprentice could enter practice or he might seek further medical training abroad, if he had the means. Edinburgh University was the favorite of American students and conferred the degree of Baccalaureate in Medicine after completion of the medical course. To receive the degree of Doctor of Medicine, a thesis must be defended at a later date.

The medical school in Edinburgh was the mecca of American students. A letter written by Samuel Bard to his father in New York in May, 1765, describes the trials of the examined student.

"...DOCTrs. Monro senior and junior with DOCTr Cullen were my private TRYALS, my Examinators. My good friend DOCTr. Hope publickly impugned my Thesis. To all of them I consider myself as much obliged for their behaviour upon these occasions in which altho they kept up the strictness of Professors, they never lost sight of the politeness of gentlemen, "The manner of my examinations was as follows: on the first I had not the most distant hint what was to be the subject of my Tryals and went on trembling, and DOCTr. Cullen after desiring me to sit down and began my Examination by asking me some general definitions as, Quid est Medicinae and so on. They then asked me some questions on the structure of the stomach and alimentary canal, thence made a digression to the Diseases (of them), examined me upon the colic Illeus, then Diagnostick and methods of Cure; then DOCTr. Monro junior asked me to distinguish bet. Illeus and Inflammation, some physiological questions upon Pulse in

This Indenture Witnesseth.

That John Rhea Barton late of Lancaster, in the State of Pennsylvania by and with the consent of his Father William Barton, hath put himself Apprentice, and by these presents doth voluntarily and of his own free will and accord put himself apprentice to Samuel Coates and Lawrence Seckel, two of the managers of the Pennsylvania Hospital, duly appointed by a Board of the said Managers a Committee for this purpose, and after the manner of an Apprentice to serve the said Samuel Coates and Lawrence Seckel their Successors and Assigns from the date of these Presents, to the tenth day of July eighteen hundred and eighteen, which will complete the full term of five Years from the day upon which he entered the Hospital on trial, during all which time; the said Apprentice his said Masters faithfully shall serve, their Secrets keep, and their lawful commands every where obey— He shall do no damage to his said Masters, nor see it done by others, without telling his said Masters have notice thereof: He shall not waste the goods of his said masters, nor lend them unlawfully to any: He shall not commit fornication, nor contract matrimony within the said term: He shall not play at Cards, dice nor any other unlawful game, whereby his said masters may have damage:— with his own goods, or the goods of others without license from his said Masters, he shall neither buy nor sell. He shall not absent him self day nor Night, from his Masters Service

Copy of an indenture for John Rhea Barton on becoming a medical apprentice in 1814.

The Indenture of John Rhea Barton on becoming a Medical Apprentice in 1814

This Indenture Witnesseth

That John Rhea Barton late of Lancaster in the State of Pennsylvania by and with the consent of his Father, William Barton, has put himself apprentice and by these presents doth voluntarily and of his own free will and accord put himself apprentice to Samuel Coates and Lawrence Sechel, two of the Managers of the Pennsylvania Hospital, duly appointed by a Board of said Managers a Committee for this purpose, and after the manner of an apprentice to serve the said Samuel Coates and Lawrence Sekel Such affors and assigns from the date of these Presents to the tenth day of July, Eighteen Hundred and Eighteen, which will complete the full time of five years from the date upon which he entered the Hospital on trial, during all of which time the said Apprentice his said Masters faithfully shall serve, their secrets keep, and their lawful command every way obey. He shall do no damage to his said Masters, nor see it done by others without telling his said Masters have noticed thereof. He shall not commit fornication not contract matrimony within the said term. He shall not play at cards, dice nor any other unlawful game whereby his said Masters may have damage: — with his own goods or the goods of others without license from his said Masters he shall neither buy or sell. He shall not absent himself day or night from his Masters Service.

Inflammation, the causes of Intussusceptio in the Intestines and the method of Cure in both these diseases. This ended my first examination which lasted about 45 minutes.

"My next Tryal was writing Commentaries upon two of Hippocrates' aphorisms and defending them. Lastly, I was publickly in Hall to defend my Thesis. During all these Tryals my Exercises were written in Latin and I was obliged to defend them in the same language...."

Early in the eighteenth century the medical school at Edinburgh forged ahead as the premier place to study in Britain and perhaps in Europe. It broke the shackles binding the teaching of medicine to Galen and metaphysical observations. William Cullen, the professor of physic, also broke tradition by lecturing in English, although the thesis for the medical degree still was to be delivered in Latin. Three generations of the Monro family in anatomy and surgery, and the work of Cullen in medicine brought fame to the institution. Benjamin

Bell, the author of the multivolume textbook of surgery, used in America, and Joseph Black, chemist and discoverer of carbon dioxide, emhanced the reputation of the school and also attracted students from America.

Admission requirements were liberalized and demanded a knowledge of natural history, botany and a general examination. Courses included anatomy, surgery, chemistry, pharmacy, theory and practice of physic, and clinical lectures at the Royal Infirmary. In 1783 the formal course included three years of study with at least one year in the infirmary. Three months before being examined for a bachelor's degree in medicine, the student had to pass an examination on literary knowledge and medical preparedness.[178] After receiving the Baccalaureate in Medicine, the student was to develop and defend his thesis for which he was granted a Doctorate of Medicine.

Other universities in Britain granted degrees for minimal achievement. At Aberdeen and St. Andrews, medical degrees were given with a payment of a fee and two recommendations of character. Oxford and Cambridge remained bridled with ancient studies and required seven years of literary study and a degree of Master of Arts before admission to the school of medicine. Once enrolled in the school of medicine, teaching followed the precepts of Galen, Paralcelsus and medieval physicians.

The American students in Edinburgh were hard-working and diligent and did well in their studies. They grouped together for study and recreation. During mornings they attended lectures, many in Latin, and took copious notes. Afternoons were spent attending lectures or revising notes. Lectures began at 8:00 a.m. and lasted until 7:00 p.m., but not all students attended each lecture. They also found time to attend clinical demonstrations and surgery at the infirmary, and applied such knowledge by dissecting animals in their quarters. Once a week the Americans would meet to discuss their progress.

Frequently they gathered together in their free hours, comparing the university medicine to which they were exposed to the low standards they remembered in America. Hunter, Fothergill, Cullen and other medical teachers encouraged them to return to America and reshape American medicine. The Virginia Medical and Anatomical Club resolved to bring back to their homeland the highest ethical standards; they would practice medicine only, sell no drugs and perform no surgery, completing the separation of physician, surgeon and apothecary. On their return they quickly learned that the rural American scene would permit no such separation. The Virginians as students drafted a letter to the Virginia Council and the House of Burgesses requesting legislation to prevent unqualified doctors from practicing.

John Morgan, William Shippen and Arthur Lee planned how they would start a medical school on their return which would be based on the Edinburgh model. After a medical faculty was added to the College of Philadelphia through the efforts of Morgan in 1765, he crusaded for laws disqualifying doctors without an educational background. He proposed a national medical society, all of whose members would have a degree granted by a national American College of Physicians, with licensing power throughout America. State's rights, local politics, and regional rivalries quickly put an end to such visionary plans.[179]

Socially, the students were often invited to the homes of the Edinburgh townspeople who were eager to listen to stories of America.[180] On their return to America they were in demand as guests to talk about their experiences, the political climate, styles of dress, and whatever was new in the mother country.

The College of Philadelphia was already functioning, having been established in 1751 through the efforts of Benjamin Franklin, and seemed receptive to the idea of a medical faculty. Morgan convinced the trustees of the college that a medical school was necessary and in May, 1765, on the opening of the school, he addressed the trustees, faculty and the general public.

In this talk, Morgan stated why a medical school was necessary, the prerequisites for entrance, the structure of the courses, and the faculty; why it was necessary to recruit eminent practitioners in the community; and the place of a hospital in medical training. Morgan also suggested that there be a division between medicine and surgical practice and pharmacy. In 1768 the first

A pass issued to a medical student permitting him to attend a lecture.

medical degrees were granted in America; these were Baccalau-reates in Medicine awarded to ten students following the system of Edinburgh. Three years later four graduates defended their theses and were granted the degree Doctors of Medicine.

In 1790 the Baccalaureate degree was discontinued and all graduates received the M.D. degree. Morgan failed to enlist the support of Shippen, who was in the audience when Morgan delivered his opening address, speaking of him in a patronizing manner, stating that his lectures were "...not——at all a collegiate undertaking."[181] This was the basis for a lifelong enmity between the two which had dire consequences later in the leadership of the medical department of the Continental army during the Revolutionary War.

Morgan emphasized the necessity of a hospital to be associated with the medical school. Pennsylvania Hospital in Philadelphia served such a purpose and was used by staff members to do bedside teaching to the medical students. It was divided into two sections: the Hospital was for ill patients, while the Bettering House was the almshouse. The Reverend Manasseh Cutler accompanied Benjamin Rush on July 14, 1787, on rounds with the students and gives us an interesting account.

> "Dr. Rush then began his examination of the sick attended by these gentlemen which, I judge to be about 20 or 30. We entered the upper chamber of the sick which is the leg of the T. It is a spacious room finely ventilated with numerous large windows on both sides. There are two tiers of beds with their heads toward the walls and a chair and small table between them. The room was exceedingly clean and nice and bedding appeared to be of good quality, and the most profound silence and order were preserved upon the doctor entering the room. There were only women and about 40 in number. Dr. Rush makes his visits with a great deal of formality. He is attended by the attending Physician who gives him an account of everything material since he saw them last, and by the Apothecary of the Hospital who minutes his prescriptions. In every case worthy of notice, he addresses the young physicians, points out its nature, the probable tendency and the reason for the mode of treatment which he prescribes."[182]

During the war the school closed, and when it reopened it had a new competing school, the University of Pennsylvania with which it merged.

In 1768 Kings' College in New York City established a medical school, later renamed Columbia College and then The College of

Physicians and Surgeons. This was followed by the medical schools at Harvard in 1782 and Dartmouth in 1797.

Samuel Bard returned from Edinburgh to practice in New York City. He delivered the commencement address at Kings' College on May 16, 1769, and said:

> "...explain to you the weighty duties of your Profession.... A Profession of which Integrity and Abilities will place you among the most useful.... Ignorance and Dishonesty will place you among the most Pernicious Members of Society. ...that your labours have no end...."

He recommended the writings of Sydenham, Boerhaave, Whytt, Huxham and Pringle; and advised the graduating class to continue learning as they practiced. They were to respect the theories of the ancients but to question them. They must practice tenderness to their patients but not to buoy up the hopes of a dying man with groundless expectations and to attend the poor without compensation.

The College of Physicians and Surgeons again requested Bard to give the commencement address fifty years later; on April 6, 1819, he stated,

> "The great error in our system of Education is that we are too much in a hurry. Our graduates are so young that they have not acquired the prudence and knowledge to govern their conduct. Among ignorant and barbarous nations, medicine has been connected with religion involving mystery and superstition. In medical science...one must see and hear and feel for himself...the hue of the complexion and the feel of the skin, the luster and languor of the eyes, the throbbing of the pulse, and the

palpitations of the heart, the quickness and ease of respiration and the tone and tremor of the voice."

The educational texts of American doctors and treatment in America was similar to that in Europe. The seven-volume surgical text of Benjamin Bell of the Edinburgh staff was for many years the standard and authoritative surgical reference. Bell was the first of a long line of scientific surgeons that made Edinburgh the medical center of Europe as well as America. Bell's text was condensed into a single volume by Nicholas Waters in America, and published in Philadelphia in 1791.[183]

The books of Sydenham, Cheselden, Monro, Heberden, and Fothergill from England were popular as well as the treatises of LeDran and Desault in France.

John Jones, professor of surgery at Kings' College in New York, wrote the first surgical textbook in America. This was an instructional course for military surgeons in 1775, entitled, *Plain and Concise Remarks on the Treatment of Wounds and Fractures*.[184] Jones' book is a resume of the texts in use at that time in Europe. Benjamin Rush, in 1790, published a system of medicine widely used in America.[185]

John Hunter's experimental notes were probably not available in America, but American doctors in London sought out Hunter to attend his lectures and many became his personal friends. His course of lectures, delivered in 1785, was taken in shorthand by James Parkinson, who later described the paralytic condition known by his name. These notes were published much later and entitled *Hunterian Reminiscences*.[186] Sir Percival Pott also entertained and taught young American doctors in London and remained a lifelong friend of John Jones, exchanging case reports and notes on surgical advances.

Lectures in anatomy and surgery were occasionally available to American students and physicians. The applicant would purchase a ticket permitting him to attend the series. In 1730 Thomas

Cadwalader of Philadelphia is on record for delivery of such a lecture series. William Hunter, relative of John Hunter, having settled in Rhode Island gave a series of anatomical lectures between 1754 and 1756. In Philadelphia in 1762 William Shippen lectured on anatomy and midwifery and repeated the course again in 1763 and 1764. Shippen soon afterwards became the first professor of surgery at the College of Philadelphia and John Bard lectured in anatomy in New York.

John Warren, brother of Joseph who was killed in the Battle of Bunker Hill, was medical director of the Continental Army Hospital in Cambridge in 1775 and early 1776, and gave a series of anatomical lectures in 1780 and 1781 which just preceded the foundation of Harvard Medical School.

At the onset of the War for Independence in 1775, the American Colonies stretched along the Atlantic seaboard from Maine to Georgia, extending westward several hundred miles. Three million Americans were served by about 3,000 physicians, of whom 400 had obtained medical degrees, the rest being trained through an apprenticeship. In addition, an unknown number of healers practiced. Between 1749 and 1800, 117 American doctors graduated from Edinburgh and perhaps another 100 took some courses but did not get a degree. Physicians returning to America with degrees also attended medical schools in Paris, Rouen, Leyden, Bonn, and Vienna. The first American doctor with a degree from Edinburgh was John Moultrie, who returned to South Carolina in 1749.

Many of the Americans attending medical schools in Europe "walked the wards" of St. Bartholomew's and Guy's hospitals in London after graduation, sharpening their clinical skills in a sort of internship.

* * * * * *

Most doctors were trained as apprentices, but healers, quacks, and patent medicine salesmen who adopted the title of doctor and conducted a medical practice with no training or aptitude and little regard for their patients continued. Dr. Alexander Hamilton, traveling about America in 1744, described an incident he encountered in Huntington, Long Island.

While Dr. Hamilton was awaiting his dinner in the local tavern, a band of politicians "...in short jackets and trowsers trooped into the dining room. Among the rest was a fellow with a worsted cap and great black fists. They stiled him doctor...he had been a shoemaker in town and was a notable fellow at his trade, but happening two years ago to cure an old woman of a pestilent mortal disease, he thereby acquired the character of a physician, was applied to from all quarters and finding the practise of physick a more profitable business than cobbling, he laid aside his awls and leather, got himself some gallipots and instead of cobbling of soals fell to cobbling of human bodies."

When Hamilton visited New England, he couldn't abide the Boston firebrand doctor, William Douglass, to whom he was introduced. Hamilton was appalled when Douglass tore apart the most respected textbook of surgery by Heister and then damned the leading physician and teacher in Europe, Boerhaave. Douglass wrote a thesis critical of Boerhaave and was pleased to note how Boerhaave was nettled. Hamilton was reminded of the response of a mastiff to a snarling lap dog and wrote of Douglass, "He is only a cynicall mortall so full of his own learning that any other man is not current with him. There are in Boston a group of half learned priggs to who Douglass is an oracle."[187]

There were many patients requiring medical attention. Most deaths were due to bacterial infections, with a high infant mortality. Only a few in the population reached the advanced age when most cancers and heart disease posed a threat.[188]

CHAPTER FIVE

THE DOCTOR AS MILITARY SURGEON
IN THE COLONIAL PERIOD

Warfare has always advanced surgery. Technical prowess improves when treating large numbers of casualties, and the results of different types of treatment can be compared. Many surgeons working together discuss their ideas, trade experiences, and when the results of different treatment are followed and evaluated, new underlying principles surface which pass from surgeon to surgeon, hospital to hospital and into the surgical literature.

At the beginning of World War I, in 1914, there was no consensus how to treat battle wounds. Some wounds were tightly closed with sutures, some simply cleansed and left open to slowly heal. Other wounds were left open initially and closed at a later time. It soon became evident that the tightly closed wound did poorly, the patient becoming septic and toxic. Gangrene and amputation resulted. Soldiers whose wounds were cleansed with removal of dead tissue, and the wound left open to be closed later, fared better. The lesson was well learned, for when World War II began, it was the official medical edict to leave wounds open with a few exceptions such as those of the face.

Before the fourteenth century, military surgeons dealt only with wounds caused by lances, spears, swords, knives, arrows, and blunt instruments. Gunpowder forever changed the strategy and tactics of warfare, and also the problems of wound treatment. Not only were the types of wounds different, but the number of casualties increased exponentially. Wounds were now caused by musket and pistol balls and whatever could be thrust down the muzzle of a cannon, whether cannon balls, segments of chains, metallic debris and even stones. Wounds from swords and bayonets continued to occur.

The first recorded use of gunpowder was in a British military operation at Crecy, France, in 1338. Surgeons were now confronted for the first time with the problem of retained metal in the wound. The number of wounded and killed shot upwards and the severe infections and tissue damage that resulted convinced surgeons that gunpowder itself was a toxic substance. Attempts at detoxification were by hot oil or the cautery applied locally to the wound site, and bleeding of the casualty to remove the spreading effects of the toxin.

In Europe and in America the treatment of battlefield wounds was influenced by the writings of Henri LeDran,[189] Baron Van Swieten[190], Benjamin Bell[191] and, especially, by Ambroise Paré. Paré (1510-1590), chief surgeon to Charles IX of France, spent much of his life treating the wounded in many campaigns. His battlefield observations were the basis for his widely acclaimed book on wound treatment in 1545, *L'Onzieme Livre Traictant des Playes Faictes par Auquebus et Autres Baton à Feu*.[192] His treatment of wounds, like those of other military surgeons of the period, was to pour hot oil in the wound after bleeding was controlled either by ligature or the cautery. In this book he describes a fortuitous experiment: "At last my supply of oil ran out, and I was obliged to use in its place a digestive of yolk of eggs, oil of roses, and turpentine. That night I could not sleep with thinking that I might find the wounded who had been deprived of oil, dead from poisoning. Beyond all my hopes... I found they were feeling little pain and were without any inflammation...others who had the oil had a fever and suffered."[194]

Paré disproved the toxic nature of gunshot wounds stating that they were simply a severely crushed wound. If such wounds were not toxic, the hot oil could be forgotten, and for bleeding greater reliance could be placed on ligation of a vessel rather than burning it with a cautery: Every effort was to be made to avoid inflicting further damage to the tissues.

In spite of the searing and tissue destruction in the wound, the pain borne by the wounded, and the stench arising from the burned flesh, some good was lost by abandonment of the oil and the cautery; the partial sterilization of the wound. The gain was greater than the loss, but some early surgeons without knowing the reason observed the loss of this sterilizing effect. Peter Lowe in England in 1529, discussing old wounds with recurrent hemorrhage, stated, "The ligature for hemorrhage when there is not suppuration present; when it is, the cautery."[194]

Paré also wrote about avoiding amputation if possible, delaying it to observe the state of the patient and his course, advising amputation only when the patient presented with a fever. Paré's teaching regarding amputations has been periodically forgotten during the conflicts of the next several hundred years. Sir Percival Potts in England during the early 18th century vigorously recommended early amputation for an open wound of the extremity. In America, during the War of Independence, a more conservative approach was observed and early amputations rarely done. During the American Civil War it again became very popular as a battlefield operation to be done directly after injury.

* * * * * *

With the beginning of hostilities in 1775, the Colonial American doctor must now be transformed to a military surgeon. Of the 3500 physicians in America, about 1400 served with the military forces, some for the entire war, others for a single battle or campaign; some with the Continental army, others with the provincial militias. Two medical schools had graduated about fifty doctors in America. About 300 doctors had received training in Europe, while the remaining doctors had acquired their medical education as apprentices. Early in the war no specific qualifications or examinations were required, but there were exceptions. The Massachusetts militia required doctors to pass an examination soon after the Battle of Bunker Hill in 1775. It was not until much later that medical warrants in the Continental army required a qualifying examination.

In order to master the surgical skills needed in warfare, the doctor depended on surgical texts available in America. The most authoritative surgical text available was the seven-volume work of Benjamin Bell of Edinburgh. To those Americans who studied at Edinburgh, this was a familiar work and it was later condensed into a single volume by Benjamin Waters of Philadelphia.[195] Some American doctors had experienced war surgery sixteen years before in the battles against the French. The Continental Congress had established a Hospital Department after Bunker Hill but training in the treatment of wounds was not provided by the Hospital Department or any of the provincial governments.

It is at this critical period that we encounter John Jones, M.D., the first professor of surgery at Kings' College in New York. Jones recognized the urgent need to educate and inform American doctors in the state-of-the-art surgery, and particularly war surgery, as it existed in Europe. He wrote a manual of surgery addressed, "to the students

PLAIN CONCISE

PRACTICAL REMARKS

Jam! ON THE TREATMENT OF *Oliver's*

WOUNDS AND FRACTURES;

TO WHICH IS ADDED, A SHORT

APPENDIX

ON

CAMP AND MILITARY HOSPITALS;

PRINCIPALLY

Defigned for the Ufe of young MILITARY SURGEONS,

in NORTH-AMERICA.

By JOHN JONES, M. D.
Proeffor of Surgery in King's College, New-York.

NEW-YORK:
by JOHN HOLT, in Water-Street, near the
Coffee-Houfe.

M,DCC,LXXV.

Title page of John Jones' book, the first American textbook of Surgery.

and young practitioners in surgery through all America." The manual was written in 1775, six months after the first clashes between the Americans and British at Lexington and Concord.[196]

Jones reveals his sentiments in the preface of this work.

> "The present calamitous situation of this once happy country in a peculiar manner demands the aid and assistance of every virtuous citizen; and though few men are possessed of those superior talents which are requisite to heal such mighty evils, yet every man has it in his power to contribute something towards so desirable an end; and if he cannot cure the fatal disease of his unfortunate country, it will at least afford him some consolation to have poured a little balm into her bleeding wounds."[197]

The second edition of Jones' book was published in Philadelphia in 1776 and included the appendix on Camp and Military Hospitals "designed for the use of young military and naval surgeons in North America."

The third edition was also published in Philadelphia in 1795, and this edition includes a short account of the life of the author by James Mease, M.D.[198]

The book is presented as an instructional course, but not to just anyone. Jones wanted only men of character to be involved in military surgery and we find among his many references the moral and ethical conduct necessary to qualify as a good surgeon..."the proper requisites of which respectable character, are only to be found in a liberal education furnishing every means of acquiring that knowledge which must be ripened by experience and graced by the practice of attention, tenderness and humanity." He was admired by his students, whom he inspired, but "admonished them to despise the servile conduct of those who consider the profession as worthy of

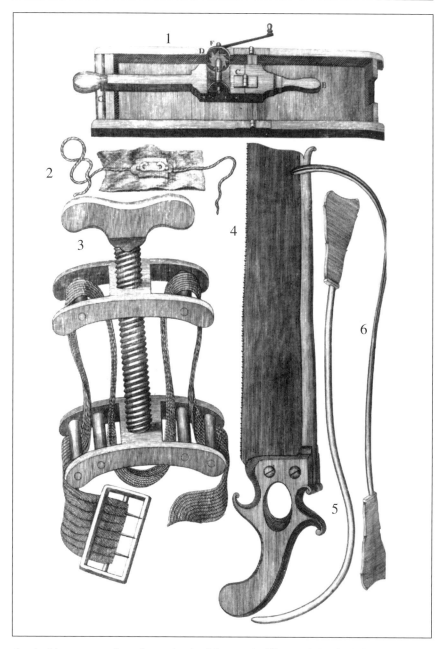

Surgical instruments from the textbook of Surgery by Waters. 1. A winch for reducing dislocations. 2. A tie for lower arm fractures. 3. A screw tourniquet. 4. An amputation saw. 5 & 6. Sounds to palpate bladder stones.

cultivation only in proportion to the emoluments which it yields."

Jones was well qualified for his position as teacher to the doctors of North America, having preceded the many American doctors who in this century and the centuries to follow completed their studies by a tour of Europe. He served an apprenticeship under Thomas Cadwalader of Philadelphia to whom his 'Remarks' are dedicated. He traveled to London, attending the lectures of John Hunter and McKenzie at St. Bartholomew's Hospital. Here he also studied under Sir Percival Potts, with whom he established a lasting friendship.

He was awarded an M.D. degree in France at the University of Rheims in 1751 and afterward worked on the wards of the Hôtel de Dieu, the enormous charity city hospital in Paris, studying under the renowned French surgeons, LeCat and LeDran. Next, on to Leyden, and finally, Edinburgh, then emerging as the center of scientific medicine. When he returned to America, he settled in New York and was appointed first professor of surgery at Kings' College.

He volunteered for service with the British during the French and Indian War in 1758. An interesting story is told of him during this enlistment, showing how widespread was his fame. In a battle with the French in upper New York State, the commander of the French force, General D'Ecaux, was dangerously wounded. He did not allow the French surgeons to treat him, but came to Jones and requested and received treatment.

With the colonies at war with Britain, Jones remained a steadfast patriot, refusing to practice in the cities occupied by the enemy. After the battle of Long Island, the British used New York as their base of operations, under General Clinton, for the remainder of the war. At that time, Jones left the city to practice in the surrounding countryside, ignoring the repeated invitation of the British commander to return to the city and continue his practice. True to his ideals, he would not accumulate wealth while the country was ravaged.

He entered the Medical Department of the Army, but his asthma, from which he suffered most of his life and which contributed to his death, forced him to leave. After leaving his military post and after the war, he settled in Philadelphia and was on the staff of the Pennsylvania Hospital and the Philadelphia Dispensary.

All of these texts on wounds recommended early operation on battle casualties, with enlargement of the wound to remove embedded metal, clothing, and debris whenever possible. The wound was usually left open or partly closed with bandages or tape. If the wound included a joint cavity, there was no hope of avoiding a violent septic reaction, and death was certain unless an early amputation was done. Otherwise, the decision to amputate was determined by a downhill course with increasing toxicity, or if the limb was so mangled that there was no hope of future function, at which time a prompt amputation became necessary.

Fractures incurred in the field of battle were to be supported by splints, and skillfully bound with bandages so the wound could be dressed without disturbing the fracture alignment. Sickness, not battlefield wounds, caused over 90% of the deaths in the American army.

It is unfortunate that an instructional manual on sanitation and the prevention of disease similar to Jones' book on surgery was not written and addressed to the military doctors when the conflict began. It was not that this information was unknown, the truth is, it was ignored. Such a book should also have been required reading for the general and field staffs. Had such information been available and implemented by command, thousands of lives would have been saved, the war more rapidly concluded, and military success so much greater that the United States might now include Canada.

Such a manual would include the tested information already published by Pringle, Surgeon General of the British army, in his book, *Observations on the Diseases of the Army*, first published in 1752.[199] Donald Monro reinforced Pringle's conclusions in his book, *An Account of the Diseases Most Frequent in Military Hospitals in Germany*, published in 1764.[200] Van Swieten's *The Diseases Incident to Armies*, translated into English, was published in 1776.[201] Richard Brocklesby, another Surgeon General of the British army, also publishd his experiences with disease in the British army.

The message so forcibly repeated in these books discussed the importance of dry clothing, frequently washed. Scavenging clothing from the dead on the field of battle or from the piles of clothing of patients dying in the hospital was strictly forbidden. Campsites should be on elevated ground and dead animals and garbage were not to accumulate around camps. Straw issued for bedding was to be frequently changed, and burned when used by a sick soldier. Water was to be mixed with wine or vinegar for purification. Soldiers were commanded to wash their face and hands and comb their hair; bathing was to be done once weekly. Proper exercise, limitation of spirituous liquor and a diet with good bread, more vegetables, and less meat was recommended. Pringle wrote regarding soldiers, "....the prevention of disease depends...on such orders as shall appear to be unreasonable to him or what he must necessarily obey."

General hospital overcrowding was to be avoided by more frequent use of regimental hospitals. The beds of the hospital were to be so separated so that there was room for another bed between each two beds. Patients with wounds and ulcers were not to be next to sick patients. Smallpox and measles were to be segregated. The hospital was fumigated at intervals with the smoke of wet gunpowder. A sergeants guard was to be assigned to keep order in the hospital, and sentries posted to prevent absences and desertions and to take roll call each morning.

In contrast, the American General Hospital early in the war was overcrowded, usually dirty, many of the patients had trivial complaints and refused to return to their units. Drunkenness was rampant, supplies were stolen and no accurate account of the number of patients in the hospital was known. It was strongly suspected during the tenure of Shippen as Director General, that census figures were padded so that increased requisitions could be made. To many soldiers the hospital was a springboard for desertion.

The American general and field officers dissociated themselves from any responsibility in preventing illness or the running of a hospital. Sanitation, cleanliness, diet and the health of the troops in their command were ignored. Washington did understand the problem and consulted with Rush on several occasions.

On April 22, 1777, Benjamin Rush had published an article in the Pennsuylvania Packet under a pseudonym entitled, "To The Officers in the Army of the United States: Directions for Preserving the Health of Soldiers." Rush had met Pringle in London and Rush was also familiar with the published works of Van Swieten, Brocklesby and Monro. The article closely followed the recommendations of these men and was divided into five sections; Dress, Diet, Cleanliness, Encampments and Exercises. It was Rush's hope that this pamphlet would be reprinted. Congress recognized the value of this work and directed it to be published as an official document titled, "Directions for Preserving the Health of Soldiers. Recommended to the Consideration of the Officers of the Army of the United States."[202] In the latter years of the war, improvements in sanitation were made and sickness decreased, but most commanding officers whose responsibility was the prevention of disease failed to appreciate the importance of their role.

Rush, in a letter to Washington on May 13, 1777, requested Washington to avoid a prolonged encampment near Morristown, New Jersey, because American troops were in a weakened state from an epidemic of smallpox. Rush quoted Pringle on the increase of disease that can be expected when armies are encamped for long periods. Washington, in his reply on May 16, 1777, stated he agreed with Rush's ideas, but brought to his attention that other factors overruled Rush's request stating, "...that the more an army is collected, the better it is adapted both for the purpose of defence and offence."

In another letter to Washington, Rush, who for a brief period was a member of the Medical Committee of Congress, was apprehensive about Southern troops marching north to join Washington, and informed Washington that the commanders of these troops were to halt and the troops inoculated for smallpox before proceeding; also some of these battalions in joining Washington were to take "the upper route", to avoid Philadelphia where smallpox was epidemic.[203]

When Baron Von Steuben came to America to command American troops, he brought with him a strict Prussian code of hygiene which he had learned from Belgauer, Chief Medical Officer of the Prussian army. Late in the war General Wayne was a convert to the principles of military hygiene and cleanliness. In the orderly book over General Wayne's signature dated March 29, 1778, this statement associating cleanliness and esprit appears.

> "As there is no Greater or purer mark of discipline than Cleanliness, so there is nothing more conductive to health and spirit; it introduces a laudable pride which is substitute for almost every virtue; the General therefore, in the most pointed terms desires the officers to oblige their men to appear clean and decent at all times and upon all occasions. Even punishing that soldier that appears dirty, whether on duty or not."

General Wayne had his troops wear a feather in their hats to set them off as a distinguishing mark.[204]

When Benjamin Rush discussed problems of sickness, hygiene and hospitalization with British officers, he discovered that unlike American officers, the matter of the sick was of great concern to the British command.

Discipline in the American militias and continental army was poorly maintained, especially in the early years of the war. At Bunker Hill, Colonel Prescott gave tactical orders to the militias some of whom responded, while others just disappeared. Many units left the battleground when the cannonading from the British fleet in the harbor began. Those that remained surprised the British commander and his officers by their heroic resistance.

When Washington arrived in Cambridge in 1775, he despaired of the absence of any military discipline. Officers were addressed by their first name by those in his command. Orders from officers were disputed; the camp was filthy with no proper sanitation control. It resembled a mob rather than an army. Militias included men who grew up together as neighbors in their home community. Addressing your friend of long-standing as captain or sir was irritating.

The Massachusetts Provincial Congress, aware of the lack of discipline, and cleanliness, and the military informality of the regimental militias in Cambridge, warned Washington of the problems he was about to face and wrote him: "We would not presume to prescribe to your excellency, but supposing you would choose to be informed of the general Character of the soldiers who compose the army, beg leave to represent that the greatest part of them have not before seen service, and although naturally brave and of good understanding, yet for want of experience in military life, have but little knowledge of divers things most essential to the preservation of health and even life. The youth of the army are not possessed of the absolute necessity in their dress and lodging, continual exercise and strict temperance to preserve them from disease, frequently prevailing in camp, especially among those who from childhood have been used to a laborious life."[205]

During the siege of Boston between July 1775 and March 1776, 15% of the army of 15,000 was sick or wounded, most being sick. Washington wisely decided that military standards would have to be gradually instituted; first orders were for the units to practice drill on the parade ground. Washington also noted the disarray of the medical doctors, the antagonisms between doctors from the various state militias, and the filth and lack of organization in the hospital at Cambridge. In desperation he wrote Congress, "I have made inquiry with respect to the establishment of the hospital and find it in a very unsettled condition. There is no principal doctor or any subordination among the surgeons; of consequence disputes and contentions have arisen and must continue until it is reduced to some system. I could wish that it was immediately taken into consideration as the lives and health of both officers and soldiers so much depend upon a due regulation of this department."[206]

When asked how the medical department should be regulated Washington replied, like the British, they have years of experience. The British army had fought campaigns throughout Europe, in North America and the West Indies. Its medical arm had received the attention of the leading doctors in England, including Pringle and Brocklesby. Washington, as a young man, had fought with the British against the French and knew of their medical organization. British general hospitals were under the authority of a physician general, who administered the hospital and visited and treated the sick. The Chief Surgeon was responsible for surgery and did not receive orders from the physician for the wounded, but must obtain the consent of the physician for elective operations. There were two surgeons and eight hospital mates under the direction of the Chief Surgeon.

British flying hospitals were halfway stations linking the regimental and general hospitals in the rear. Regimental hospitals supported each regiment and their surgeons were appointed by the regimental commanders. Friction in distributing supplies between regimental and hospital surgeons was ever present, just as it was in the American forces. Purveyors were in charge of distributing supplies and received twenty-five shillings a day, physicians twenty shillings, surgeons and apothecaries ten, and mates five shillings daily. The main British hospital base during the war was in New York, where there were seven general hospitals with 3000 beds.

The reply from Congress to Washington lacked vision and understanding. It considered only the situation in Cambridge, made no provision for other hospitals in other areas or the medical needs of an army in battle. Congress responded by appointing a Director General, a chief physician, four surgeons, one apothecary, twenty surgeons mates, storekeepers, plus one nurse for every ten sick.

We have incidents reported throughout the war indicating lapses in medical discipline in the army. Benjamin Rush noted that too many soldiers were in hospitals too long, abusing their privileges by drunkenness, selling government items to the local inns in exchange for liquor, and being absent without leave. Rush wrote to General Greene, "We have in the hospital of this place soldiers, many of whom have complaints so trifling that they do not prevent them from committing daily a hundred irregularities of all kinds. The physician and surgeon of the hospital have no power to prevent or punish.... A soldier should never be suffered to exist a single hour without a sense of his having a master being impressed upon his mind.... It is no purpose to train your men to subordination in the field or camp. In one month they will lose in our hospitals the discipline of a whole year...."[207]

British hospitals were assigned details of men, commanded by a corporal to maintain strict discipline within the hospital and also a staff of sentries to prevent wandering and desertion by the inmates. In the British army the regimental commander appointed the regimental surgeon. In America also, the regimental colonel of the militias of the various colonies appointed the medical officer in each regiment, but experienced difficulty in keeping his medical officer for more than a few months. The regimental surgeon, usually a friend of the colonel, would remain with the unit as long as he was close to his village, but would resign when the unit was ordered to move to a distant area. Financial factors as well as separation from family were also responsible. The average rural doctor earned about 900 dollars a year, the town doctor about 1500 dollars a year, but the regimental surgeon was paid only about 25 dollars a month. The British regimental surgeon was paid four shillings daily.

The American regimental surgeon had little knowledge of how he was to function. The duties of the British regimental surgeon are discussed in detail by Dr. R. Hamilton, a regimental surgeon, and published in this period.[208] The regimental surgeon must attend all field exercises and remain with his unit in battle. Field officers often looked down on the regimental surgeon, failing to understand that in that era more men died in the army by disease than the lance. When the regimental general officer was understanding and generous, Hamilton writes, this attitude filters down to the lower officers and the men, and the lot of the regimental surgeon is improved.

British army discipline was necessarily strict, to ensure proper behavior and subordination in the chain of command. The regimental surgeon was also required to attend all punishments, and he was the only officer aside from the commanding officer who could commute or end a physical punishment. Anthony Gregory, of the tenth regiment of foot soldiers, was punished with 100 lashes for allowing the queue of his hair to drop off while on duty. Those wielding the whip were instructed and supervised by the surgeon to avoid the head and legs, and concentrate on the back, buttocks and shoulders. If the victim asked for a drink, the surgeon must stop the punishment and provide it. The surgeon was to examine the victim periodically; continued fainting, turning cold or failure of the pupil of the eye to react were reasons for discontinuing the punishment. The philosophy of such severe discipline and punishment is borne out by an incident in America. A British grenadier stationed in New Jersey during the war was court-martialed for striking a captain and sentenced to 1000 lashes, but the British commanding general disapproved of the sentence and sent the grenadier under guard back to England. Three days later another trooper in the same unit struck an officer. In three hours he was hanged, and there were no further incidents of insubordination in this regiment.[209]

* * * * * *

There was never any written agreement between the British and Americans on prisoner exchange or treatment of captured enemy medical officers or equipment, hospitals, care of the wounded and their disposition. This was all the more inexplicable because a precedent for the Geneva Convention's principles was established and regulated by Pringle in 1743. Pringle, when physician for the British forces under the Earl of Stair in the battle of Dettingen in Bavaria, obtained an agreement with the Duc de Noailles, the French commander, to declare military hospitals of both forces, neutral and immune sanctuaries.[210] Moreover, in the preface to his book, Pringle wrote, "It would be a right good measure in the beginning of every war to settle by a Cartel that military hospitals on both sides should be ordered as santuaries for the sick and mutually protected." One possible reason for not considering such an agreement was the British attitude toward the Americans that they were suppressing an insurrection of rebels, not fighting a national enemy.

There was a tacit understanding that medical men after capture would be returned to the enemy. This was less true of hospital equipment, which was often in short supply on both sides. Throughout the war when wounded prisoners required treatment, the enemy was invited to supply doctors to aid in their treatment. After the battle of Germantown in Pennsylvania, British surgeons were assisted by American surgeons from the College of Philadelphia.[211] American casualties from this battle required transportation to the hospital at Bethlehem for treatment.

In South Carolina, Dr. Williamson of the Continental army was permitted by General Cornwallis to treat wounded American prisoners. Americans claimed that these prisoners were originally neglected, but the British surgeon, Dr. Hayes, and eleven of his staff were severely ill and even the British casualties received no treatment. Sickness, presumably due to malaria, was so great that Cornwallis refused to establish a camp within 100 miles of the coast. At the Battle of Cowpens in South Carolina, arrangements were quickly made to exchange wounded prisoners. Special consideration was given the British surgeon, Dr. Robert Jackson, who so impressed the American command with his heroism in saving General Tarleton that although unwounded, he was permitted to return to his lines without an exchange being demanded.[212]

During the forays around Albany in 1777, at the time of Burgoyne's surrender, Jackson requested and received safe transport of his casualties to an American hospital, where British, Hessian and American doctors treated their patients side-by-side in the American hospital at Albany.

Benjamin Rush received permission to treat wounded American prisoners in the British hospital after the Battle of Brandywine in Pennsylvania. In return, Rush interceded for a British officer of the 17th regiment, Captain McPherson, an American prisoner who was wounded in the battle at Princeton, a ball penetrating his lung. The captain survived, but his recovery was slow and painful and a sea voyage recommended. Rush wrote Washington on August 30, 1777, requesting permission to allow him to go through the American lines to British-held New York City. On September fourth Washington wrote the American commandant of British prisoners to issue him a pass on his parole to New York.[213]

General Hugh Mercer was also wounded at the Battle of Princeton but was not treated with such humanity. Mercer was a distinguished American doctor who had graduated from the Medical School at Edinburgh. He elected to become a line officer rather than

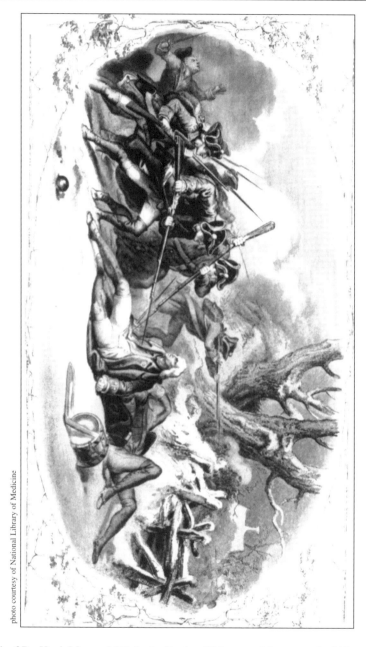

Death of Dr. Hugh Mercer, M.D. in the Battle of Princeton. Mercer received his medical degree in Edinburgh before emigrating to America at the outbreak of the war. He volunteered as a line officer rather than a Doctor, and rose to the position of a Brigadier General. He died January 12, 1776.

join the medical department. During the battle his brigade retreated, leaving the general surrounded by British troops. His horse was shot from under him; then, drawing his sword, he continued to resist until he was overwhelmed with six bayonet wounds. Unable to continue fighting, his head was then clubbed by the butt of a musket. Rush describes finding Mercer on the field of battle, barely alive.[214] "We found a number of wounded officers and soldiers belonging to both armies. Among the former was General Mercer an American, and Captain McPherson, a British officer. They were under the command of a British surgeon's mate who committed them both to me. General Mercer had been wounded by a bayonet in his belly in several places but received a stroke with the butt of a musket on the side of his head which ended his life a week after the battle."[215]

Early in the war, Congress tried to establish a Geneva-type of covenant. Dr. Huddlestone, a British surgeon, was captured by the Americans. The fate of the doctor was discussed by Congress, which ordered that Huddlestone be released and carry to his commanding officer, General Tarleton, a letter:

> "To enter into a stipulation on both sides not only to release all physicians and surgeons—but that if by the fortunes of war, the Hospital of either army should fall into the power of the other, the same substance and supplies should be afforded to the sick and wounded as if Friends: and that neither they nor the Attendants of the Hospitals should be considered or detained as Prisoners. And it is further the Opinion of the Committee that if General Tarleton should not agree to the mutual release of Surgeons, Dr. Huddlestone is to be on his Parole to return immediately thither."

This was written in the hand of Benjamin Franklin. There is no information whether Tarleton agreed or Huddlestone returned.[216]

In the darkest hours of Valley Forge in January 1778, a dispatch was delivered to Washington that helped dispel some of the gloom. The British brig *Symmetry* loaded with supplies, was captured on the Delaware River. The customs of the period demanded that the captured prize be divided among the officers; the medical men having no rank were excluded and not offered a share. They complained to Dr. John Cochran, the acting medical director, who brought the complaint to Washington, who in turn wrote to General Smallwood, who had captured the brig.

> "Since writing to you this morning on the subject of the prize Brig Symmetry, the Regulations of the Field Officers for conducting the sale and disposing of the cargo was laid before me with a letter from the regimental surgeons and mates by Dr. Cochran....
>
> "As the common guardian of the Rights of every man in this Army, I am constrained to interfere in this matter to say that by these regulations a manifest injury is intended not only for the Gentlemen in the medical line but to the whole staff..."

Washington's respect for medicine and science is again shown in another instance of the capture of this brig. He wrote to General Smallwood:

> "A few days ago I received a very polite letter from Doctor Bayes, Surgeon of the 15th British Regiment, requesting me to return him some valuable medical manuscripts taken on the Brig Symmetry. He says they are packed in a neat kind of portable library and consist of Dr. Cullen's lecture on the practice of medicine, 39 or 40 volumes, Cullen's lectures on the Institute of Medicine,

18 volumes, Anatomical Lectures, 8 volumes and Dr. Black on Chemistry, 9 volumes; the whole in octavo. If they can be found, I beg that they be sent up to me that I may return them to the Doctor. I have no other view in doing this than in showing our enemies that we do not war against sciences."[217]

Dr. Cullen of the Royal Infirmary at Edinburgh was a distinguished teacher of medicine who taught many of the Americans, who before the war traveled to Edinburgh for their medical degrees.

* * * * * *

Unfortunately the day-by-day account of military surgeons during the War of Independence was never recorded in detail. We do, however, have the journals of three doctors to describe their experiences. The military journal of Dr. Isaac Senter records the trials of the American expeditionary campaign of Colonel Arnold in his quest to capture Quebec and extend the revolution to Canada. The second journal is that of John Fish Merrick, who also accompanied troops in the Canadian campaign.[218] The third doctor to leave his journal was Dr. James Thacher, who served throughout the war.[219,220]

Isaac Senter of Londonderry, New Hampshire, studied medicine as an apprentice to Dr. Thomas Moffat, and volunteered his services, at the age of twenty-two, to the Continental army outside of Boston in the fall of 1775. The primary strategy of the newborn American army was to retake Boston from the British, but the untrained army and militias in Cambridge needed training and unification. Washington, at this stage of waiting, agreed to send two armies into Canada seeking the support of the Canadians and to urge them to join the struggle for freedom. One force was to journey from Ticonderoga up Lake Champlain to capture Montreal and then Quebec. The second force was to be a secret expedition from Cambridge by boat to the mouth of the Kennebec River in Maine; to go by boat upstream to the Chaudiere River. The two armies were to assemble before Quebec and take this almost unassailable city atop the cliffs on the St. Lawrence River.

The army against Montreal was commanded by General Schuyler, but as the result of an illness the command passed to General Montgomery. An army of 1100 men portaging up the Kennebec River and through the Maine wilderness with Senter as the surgeon was commanded by Colonel Benedict Arnold.

Dr. Senter was overwhelmed with illness in his force almost from the start. At first it was dysentery, followed by rheumatism and arthritis. Senter describes many of the men being in pitiful condition, unable to move and infested with vermin, yet he proudly states that on November 1st, after almost two months in the field, he had lost only three men. In December, with the weather turning colder, frequent portages, and marching without sufficient clothes, often shoeless, over frozen ground and on limited rations, the troops suffered from pneumonia and pleurisy as their chief complaints.

Some of the units turned back, but the more hardy continued against mounting odds in this historic march. On December 17 smallpox broke out, probably contracted from the Canadians or Indians they encountered as they entered the farm areas around Quebec. On December 18 he counted five cases and in the following days more cases were treated. Most of these New England, Pennsylvania and Virginia soldiers were from remote farms and had no immunity. Senter inoculated himself with some of the smallpox crusts from his patients on December 25.

Poised for the attack, Arnold awaited Montgomery, who had already captured Montreal but had been delayed by supply problems so that the element of surprise was lost and the city's defenders were heavily reinforced. Some of Arnold's captains refused to mount the attack, whereupon Dr. Senter volunteered to head a company. Arnold replied:

> "Dear Sir, I am obliged to you for your offer and glad to see you so spirited, but cannot consent you should take up arms as you will be wanted in the way of your profession. You will please to prepare dressings, etc., and repair to the main guard house at two o'clock in the morning with an assistant, B. Arnold, Col."[221]

In a blinding snowstorm on the last evening of 1775 the two armies struggled up the cliffs toward Quebec. Senter was receiving some wounded in the hospital and at daylight, January 1st, Colonel Arnold was brought to the hospital supported by two soldiers, hopping on his sound leg. A piece of musket ball had entered the outer side of his leg about midway and in an oblique course passed between the tibia and fibula and lodged in the calf muscles. Senter examined him, stating, "I easily discovered it and extracted it. Colonel Ogden then came in wounded in the left shoulder."[222]

News came to the hospital that General Montgomery had been killed leading his forces, that his troops were retreating and the enemy had come out of the fort and were advancing toward the hospital, which also was a command post. There was no immunity at that time, or at any time during the war, nor a covenant for the protection of hospitals and their patients and personnel.

Those patients that could walk were evacuated. Arnold would not surrender and he ordered his pistols loaded and his sword laid across his bed, stating he would kill as many as possible if they entered. Muskets were passed out to other patients. Fortunately, the British didn't advance far enough to take the hospital.

The wounded Arnold, with his remaining troops, laid siege to Quebec and Senter notes in his journal under the date of January 6 that a number of officers and men inoculated themselves against smallpox which was contrary to orders. Self-inoculation, improperly done, could cause spread of the disease if the treated were allowed to mix with the troops. It could also cause a severe attack of the disease or death.

* * * * * *

John Fisk Merrick was a surgeon's mate attached to Colonel Elisha Porter's regiment, which was ordered to reinforce the armies besieging Quebec. This was a futile effort promoted by Arnold, now a general, to take Quebec. The city was now heavily reinforced and additional British troops and naval support were on the way.

Merrick left his home at Wilbrahim, Massachusetts, on April 22, 1776, and recorded his travels north on Lake Champlain as far as Chambly, near St. Johns. Smallpox and dysentery broke out soon after the troops moved and dogged the regiment continuously. At Chambly, General Arnold ordered physicians to inoculate the troops against smallpox. Almost immediately, the order was countermanded by General John Thomas who threatened that anyone found inoculating would be put to death. Thomas himself developed smallpox and died shortly afterward.

Defeated, the regiment retreated south on the lake. Merrick describes how he treated his patients, seeing them daily, dressing their sores and recording their deaths. Starvation and desertion were rampant. The few remaining unaffected soldiers and Merrick himself rowed the patients to Crown Point and he finally delivered them to the surgeon at Fort George.[223]

The siege of Quebec continued to May with smallpox taking an increasing toll. Senter was inoculating troops, a regiment at a time in both armies. At this time British warships and marines arrived to reinforce Quebec and the Americans withdrew to Montreal, then to St. Johns and later back to Lake Champlain.

The entire American campaign into Canada fell apart because of smallpox. General Sullivan wrote, "The raging of the smallpox deprived of whole regiments in a few days." Yet the British forces remained unscathed, possibly because there was not any contact between the two forces during the siege.

John Adams on the fourth of July, 1776, wrote, "Our army at Crown Point is an object of wretchedness enough to fill a human mind with horror;—displaced, defeated, and discontented, dispirited, diseased, naked, undisciplined, eaten up with vermin, no clothes, no beds, no medicines, no victuals, but salt pork and flour....It would make a heart of stone melt to hear the moans and see the distress of the sick and dying."[224] Driven by desperation the troops took to inoculating themselves with pus from the dried scabs of smallpox victims.

In spite of lack of food and munitions, mounting disease and desertions, and indescribable physical hardships those who finally fought before Quebec were praised by Congress, the Army Corps and even the British military.

* * * * * *

Infantrymen of all nationalities on the battlefields of America during the Revolutionary War were provided with a musket and an attached bayonet. The musket had a smooth bore barrel, and in the case of the British musket, projected a three-quarter inch lead ball with accuracy a distance of about 100 yards.[225] Loading was an onerous task, requiring putting powder into the muzzle followed by the ball which must be rammed snugly against the powder. The firing mechanism required a steel hammer to strike a piece of flint which showered sparks on some powder in the pan which ignited. Some of the flame flared into the touchhole of the barrel and ignited the main powder charge. A skillful musketeer might fire such a weapon five times a minute, but most could not equal this. The slow rate of firing while defending a position allowed rapid advancement of an enemy column and frequent hand-to-hand conflict depending on bayonets and swords.

Rifle companies of sharpshooters used the more accurate rifle, the inner barrel of which was rifled. The ball was wrapped in oil cloth which allowed a tighter fit and a greater muzzle velocity, carrying the ball accurately up to 200 yards. The weapon was so long that it couldn't be attached to a bayonet. Riflemen were therefore supplied with long knives and tomahawks for infighting.

American artillery included guns, howitzers and mortars, many captured from the British or cast in France.

Musketeers and riflemen suffered frequent burns about the hands and face from flashback from the pan when too much powder was used and also suffered burns from residual unburnt powder in the muzzle. Artillery men were injured by premature explosions from smoldering wadding after the gun fired. Casualties were few from artillery in land warfare but in a naval engagement, where great concentrations of cannons fought close range duels, most casualties were from cannon fire. Sharpshooters in the rigging also took their toll.[226,227]

* * * * * *

In 1777, the British decided upon a strategic plan to cut New England, the hotbed for independence, off from the rest of the colonies. A British force, assembled in Canada under General Burgoyne, would travel south on Lake Champlain to Lake George and Albany and be joined with a second force under General Howe from New York traveling up the Hudson River Valley. Like so many other grand plans of the British, the commanders failed to cooperate, and Howe, instead of advancing north to meet Burgoyne, went south to take Philadelphia.[228]

Meanwhile, Burgoyne's force, now near Saratoga, was in a precarious position. His right flank was crushed by the Americans under General Arnold, his left flank under attack by General Stark, and his rear open to attack by American forces threatening Fort Ticonderoga. After a series of battles in which his forces suffered heavy casualties, Burgoyne withdrew, leaving his dead on the field.

* * * * * *

James Thacher applied as surgeon to the Continental army at age 21, in 1775, and describes being one of sixteen surgeons asked to take a qualifying examination, on this occasion. Thacher writes of inoculating troops against smallpox using smallpox crusts. Later he served at Ticonderoga and Saratoga and was on active duty during the siege of Yorktown. After his retirement he wrote *The American Medical Biography*, which sketched the careers of 168 prominent doctors in America and which was published in 1828.[229]

Under the date of October 24, 1777, Thacher writes that the hospital at Albany was filled with 1000 patients including officers and men from the American, British and Hessian forces. The Dutch Church as well as several surrounding houses were requisitioned as the hospital. Thirty American surgeons and mates worked from morning until late at night dressing wounds, amputating limbs, and trepanning fractured skulls.[230] Operations were performed on soiled wooden tables contaminated with old blood, pus, feces and urine. The surgeon in a blood-stained apron stored his suture material in his lapels. The hands of the surgeon were unwashed and bloodied from handling previous casualties.

Although the hospital was American, British surgeons treated wounded British prisoners and Hessian surgeons treated their troops. Thacher expresses admiration for the skill and dexterity of the British surgeons, but considers the Hessian surgeons clumsy and oblivious to suffering.

Working in the hospital at Albany, Thacher wrote:

"The wounded and sick of our army and the enemy who have fallen into our hands, are crowding into our hospitals and require our constant attention. A considerable number of the officers and men wounded in the late battle have been brought here to be accommodated in our hospital. Several of these unfortunate but brave men received wounds of a very formidable and dangerous nature and many of them must be subjected to capital operations, (amputations or trepanning of the skull for head wounds).

"Here is a fine field for professional improvement; amputating limbs, trepanning fractured skulls and dressing the most formidable wounds have familiarized my mind to scenes of woe. A military hospital is peculiarly calculated to afford samples of affliction and to interest our sympathies and commiserations. If I turn from beholding mutilated bodies, mangled limbs, and bleeding incurable wounds, a spectacle no less revolting is presented of miserable objects languishing under afflicted diseases."[232]

Some of the soldiers had wounds which had been neglected and which were covered with maggots. Thacher applied Tincture of Myrrh which quickly cleared the wounds.

"It is my lot to have twenty wounded men committed to my care."

Thacher was sentimentally moved surveying the carnage about him when he wrote:

> "No parent, wife or sister to wipe the tears of anguish from their eyes or to soothe the pillow of death. They look up to their physician as their only earthly friend and comforter."

It was in this hospital that General Benedict Arnold was a patient with a musket ball wound of the leg, his second injury of the war. He was first wounded in the leg by a musket ball which was removed at the American hospital in the attack on Quebec. When Arnold was wounded this second time, he came under Thacher's care. Thacher wrote:

> "I watched with the celebrated General Arnold whose leg was badly fractured by a musket ball while engaging with the enemy.... He is very peevish under his misfortunes and required all my attention during the night."

Thacher does not relate the treatment of General Arnold, but he fully recovered.

The hospital at Albany was under the command of Dr. Jonathan Potts. Potts had studied at Edinburgh, but did not remain there long enough to get his degree which he finally received from the College of Philadelphia as a member of the first graduating class. His ability to command a multinational group of doctors and to expeditiously treat a heavy flow of casualties from both armies earned Potts a commendation from the Continental Congress which in a resolution passed on November 6, 1777, recognized him for his professionalism. This was one of the few occasions that the Congress singled out a doctor for high praise.[233]

The rapid influx of casualties forced Potts to institute a triage system. Sprains, dislocations and simple fractures were put on hold for treatment later. Surgeons' mates treated the numerous cases of powder burns caused by flashback from residual unburned powder in the musket pan or from the premature ignition of powder from the touchhole of a cannon.

Head injuries were on hold. If a skull was fractured or if brain damage could be ascertained, they were later trephined to release intracranial pressure. Penetrating wounds of the chest or abdominal cavities were beyond surgical treatment and were accepted as fatal. A protruding gut could be packed into the abdominal cavity and closed with a running (glover's) suture of linen or cotton. Visible bleeding vessels were ligated, but no attempt was made to repair the internal organs.

The teachings of Hunter, LeDran, and John Jones in America were followed in making a decision for an amputation. There was to be no immediate amputation unless the limb was so mangled that function was totally lost, or if the wound was through a joint; such a wound inevitably became very purulent and toxic and lead to death. Other serious wounds were to be observed and carefully followed. If the casualty was running a high fever, and was toxic, or if the beginning of mortification was noted, an amputation was indicated. The proper timing for amputations under battlefield conditions presented enormous difficulties.

On August 6, 1777, the Tryon County, New York, militia, under the command of General Nicholas Herkimer, engaged Tories and Indians protecting Burgoyne's right flank in one of the bloodiest battles of this campaign. Early in the battle, Herkimer's leg was shattered by a musket ball. "After the action, the general was taken to his own house about three miles east of Little Falls on the south bank of the Mohawk River, where his leg was amputated nine days after the battle. It is said to have been done in the most unskillful manner, the leg having been cut off square, without allowing flesh enough below the bone to cover the wound, whereby the flow of blood was with difficulty staunched."[234] Some said the amputation should have been done sooner to prevent mortification. In this instance, delay was probably the cause of death.

Wounds that were actually bleeding received first priority. If necessary a tourniquet, which was a leather belt, was placed around the limb. If the surgeon could locate the source of bleeding, a ligature of shoemaker's thread or heavy cotton was placed. At other times a styptic or cautery was used. Pressing a wad of lint into the wound would sometimes accomplish the same purpose.

Wounds were enlarged and explored with a tenaculum or the finger looking for the ball and removing it if possible. Shreds of clothing, stones, wood splinters and soil would be removed, if found. Most surgeons did not lavage the wound, but sometimes dressings soaked in wine or brandy were used to cover the wound. Turpentine would sometimes be instilled into the injured area. The wound was carefully covered with dressings to exclude air to prevent corruption. Sometimes an incision was made distant to the injury for removal of a metallic fragment, but when it proved difficult to locate the ball, the surgeon was obliged to leave it. If there was pus, no attempt was made to remove the ball. All of this surgery was done without knowledge of the existence of bacteria. It seems remarkable that any casualty survived.

The dressings remained undisturbed for two or three days. If upon removal of the dressing the limb was feverish, swollen and exquisitely painful, an incision was made in some other area to allow release of pus. Every wound must exude pus, and the surgeon termed this "laudable pus" for if the pus was draining to the exterior, the patient was not collecting a reservoir of undrained pus, which could spread and cause toxicity and death.

Later the lips of the wound were brought together by sticking plaster or even closed with a suture. The patient was supported with wine but if his course was complicated by the "hectic fever" or toxicity he might also be bled, exsanguinated as he already might be from his injury, to draw out the toxins.

Many retained musket balls caused no symptoms. LeDran accounted for this good fortune "...that is the work of nature for which we are not obliged to account for." If the wound continued to drain and a permanent suppurative tract resulted, LeDran accepted this philosophically as inevitable."[235]

If the injury had caused a fracture, the wound was to be treated in the same way. Fragments of loose bone were to be removed and the fracture ends approximated by the hand of the surgeon manipulating the ends of the bone if the wound was large enough, or in the case of small wounds by traction on the limb. Splints of wood or pasteboard were used to support the fracture. These were to be bandaged around the limb in a skillful manner so that the wound could be dressed without disturbing the fracture.

Severe head wounds were all treated with trepanning; drilling a hole in the skull to allow escape of built up pressure; blood clots and loose fragments of bone in the case of a fracture. Modern neurosurgery still employs this operation to decompress the brain.

If the chest cavity was the site of an injury it was drained of pus and blood if the wound was open, and an occlusive dressing applied. If there was a small wound of entrance, most surgeons would dress the wound and not explore the chest. If profuse hemorrhage was present from the interior of the chest cavity, treatment was by bleeding. With removal of sufficient blood, the blood pressure of the patient would fall so low that the bleeding would stop. It was hoped the damaged vessel would clot under these conditions and the clot would hold as the pressure rose later.

Abdominal wounds were not explored. This was a black box for which there was no treatment. Bleeding was controlled, if possible, through the wound entrance and if a lacerated viscus was seen it was sewn together, but the usual treatment was to repack the viscera into the cavity and tape and bandage the wound tightly, so evisceration did not recur. Most patients with abdominal wounds died within a few days.

All wounds of the spine were regarded as mortal if the spinal marrow (spinal cord) was injured. Only the surface wound was treated, not the nerve and bone structures.

During a lull in the fighting, Thacher described the admission of Captain Greg from a New York regiment who with two companions went on a pigeon shooting expedition along the Mohawk River. They blundered into an Indian ambush and all three were shot, scalped, and left for dead. The captain later became conscious and expecting to die laid his head on the chest of his dead comrade as a pillow, awaiting death. A faithful dog that had accompanied him remained close by, licking his wounds. He directed the dog to go for help and the animal, running a mile, accosted two fishermen. By "whining and piteous cries" the dog had them follow him into the woods. They feared a trap, but the dog grabbing their clothes guided them to the injured captain. Thacher describes his treatment of a scalped patient which in this case was successful, although the captain complained of his appearance.

A short distance away Burgoyne's hospital with 300 sick and wounded had to be abandoned. He sent General Gates, the American commander, a note.

> "Sir, the state of my hospital makes it more advisable to leave the wounded and sick officers whom you will find in my last camp than to transport them with the army. I recommend them to the protection which I feel I would show to an enemy in the same case."

The note was carried by Dr. John Hayes, a prominent London doctor who was left in charge of the hospital and who rode out under the protection of a white flag of truce and was escorted to Major

Wilkinson of the American army who was also a medical graduate.

Wilkinson wrote, "I accompanied him to the hospital where I found 300 men comfortably accommodated. I was introduced to the officers who occupied Sword's House and persuade myself, those of them that live, will bear in memory the hearty cheering consolation I gave them by the assurance of protection in their person and property."[236]

Hayes later informed Potts, the American surgeon in charge at Saratoga, that he had 254 casualties that should be removed to the American hospital and asked Potts to send wagons to fetch them. Later, Hayes requested litter bearers for 50 men so badly maimed, "...their wounds would not admit the motion of carts." One must admire this surgeon for the compassion he showed his patients in the face of such difficult circumstances.

* * * * * *

A number of British officers' wives who had accompanied their husbands through the lakes and forests of the primitive Northeast awaited evacuation in the Taylor Farm near Saratoga and were caring for wounded officers. Baroness Riedesel, wife of the Hessian commander, in this farmhouse wrote in her memoirs:

> "About four o'clock in the afternoon, instead of the general who was to dine with us, they brought me upon a litter poor General Fraser, mortally wounded...
>
> "The ball had gone through his bowels precisely as in the case of Major Harnage. I knew no longer which way to turn. The whole entry was filled with the sick who were suffering with the camp sickness—a kind of dysentery. I spent the whole night in this manner comforting Lady

Ackland whose husband was wounded and a prisoner; at another time looking after my children.... Early in the morning at eight o'clock, he died. At every instant wounded officers of my acquaintance arrived and the cannonade began again."[237]

After Burgoyne surrendered, Lady Ackland requested of Burgoyne a letter to the American commander, General Gates, permitting her to visit her wounded husband in the American hospital. Regarding this episode, Burgoyne wrote:

"Though I was ready to believe, for I had experienced that patience and fortitude in a supreme degree were to be found as well as every other virtue under the most tender form, I was astonished at the proposal. After so long an agitation of the spirits, exhausted not only for want of rest, but absolute want of food, drenched in rain for twelve hours, that a woman should be capable of delivering herself to an enemy, probably in the night and uncertain into what hands she might fall, appeared an effort above human virtue...a woman of the most tender and delicate frame, of the gentlest manners, habituated to the soft elegancies and refined enjoyments that attend high birth and fortune.... Her mind alone was formed for such trial."[238]

After much persuasion Burgoyne wrote the requested note to General Gates.

Lady Ackland, in the dead of night, went downriver in a boat through the battlefield swarming with night patrols and roving Indian bands. She was challenged and picked up by an American patrol and delivered to General Gates, who provided her with an escort to the hospital where she was rejoined with her husband. The

American military officers provided every courtesy to both Major Ackland and his wife during his convalescence. Several years later, back in England, he challenged another British officer to a duel after this officer made disparaging remarks about American officers and troops. Major Ackland died of wounds received from that duel.[239]

A rough idea of the nature of battle wounds seen in those who survived can be gleaned from a report of Virginia doctors examining disabled veterans who were applying for pensions at the end of the war. Most of the disabled veterans had limb wounds, usually draining infections of bones from an open fracture or amputations; some superficial head and spine wounds and some blindness were recorded. Rarely was a patient who had received a penetrating head wound or a wound of the abdominal or chest cavity alive to claim his pension.

Disputes about the proper treatment of wounds continued throughout the war. A British surgeon, Doctor Jackson, reported that war wounds would do better without enlargement or any surgical treatment. He was a physician in the Southern campaign serving with General Cornwallis who noted that militiamen wounded in Georgia, who due to the exigencies of the battle were given no treatment except a dressing to cover the wounds, healed rapidly.

At the Battle of Cowpens in South Carolina in 1781, two groups of wounded were identified. Those who received treatment "...neither got so well, so soon, with so little trouble as those who cured themselves." All were lodged in country huts. Doctor Jackson proposed laudanum, "spiritual" liquors and pouring cold water on injured limbs as the sole treatment.[240]

It was observed by another military surgeon after the Battle of Guilford in North Carolina, that when it was necessary for the army to make long forced marches, that the wounded who were carried on litters or in wagons and on horseback healed their wounds en route;

when they halted for a few days (and presumably received treatment), the wound worsened. The surgeon implied that the worsening of wounds was due to freer access to "spirituous" liquors, which could then be obtained on the stopovers.

* * * * * *

Naval warfare ranged throughout the Atlantic and the Caribbean Sea. American ships were trading with the Dutch Island of St. Eustacius and some French West Indian islands and also intercepting British ships supplying the port cities. American naval vessels attacked British shipping off the coast of England and Europe, refitting in French ports. They were aided by privateers who also took a toll on British transports.

Baron Van Swieten described treatment of war wounds in his work, *The Diseases Incident to Armies.*[241] Van Swieten was from Holland, but accepted an offer to become physician to Empress Maria Theresa in Austria, where he became chief physician to the Medical School of Vienna and was well known as a surgeon throughout Europe. His book was later translated by John Ranby, Surgeon General to the British army and excerpts from the book on *Naval Medicine* were made by William Northcote which he titled, *Extracts from the Marine Practice of Physic and Surgery for the Use of Military and Naval Surgeons in America.*[242]

Northcote discussed surgery on board naval vessels and lists equipment to be included in the medical chest of the naval surgeon. Several tourniquets, crooked needles of all sizes fully prepared with ligatures, a large quantity of lint, some mixed with flour to absorb drainage, double and single roller bandages of all sizes, needles, thread, pins, pledgets of tow, splints, bolsters, and tape to secure the splints, must all be in a state of readiness.

Instructions to the surgeon are specific. When the enemy ship is sighted, request of the captain the use of part of the ship as a surgical station. The carpenter is directed to lay a platform for the wounded over which an old sail is used as a cover and on top of which is placed seamen's bedding. "Consult with your mates and assistants so each one knows his station and duty." Request of the first officer sufficient number of hands for assistance in transporting the wounded. Collect special pursers beds for the captain and officers if they are wounded. All sickness is to be sent below to their hammocks as the platform is for wounded only.

At sea, most injuries were from cannon fire directly, or from wooden splinters or iron from the decks, masts or spars showering down on the crew. When the ships were at close range or boarded, fire from sharpshooters in the rigging, and bayonet or sword wounds contributed their share of casualties.

The surgeon attempts to remove in-driven fragments as far as possible. Probing for fragments is done sparingly and with the hand rather than an instrument which could cause more damage. Fragments that can't be readily removed are left. Small wounds are enlarged and bleeding controlled with pressure or ligation or a tourniquet. Fractures are splinted and mangled limbs or limbs with exposed joints, amputated.

As the cannonading begins, if several wounded arrive at one time, the worst injuries are to take precedence, otherwise dress the wounded as they arrive without distinction. "You should use expedition, but don't hurry." In respect to the wounded you should act as if you were entirely unaffected by their groans and complaints, but behave with caution, not rashly or cruelly, nor cause any unnecessary pain. Tourniquets are to remain in place after amputations, loosely applied, and the patient is instructed how to tighten it if bleeding starts, and he is without medical aid. The wounded are attended to make them as comfortable as possible.

In colder climates, the benumbed wounded should not immediately be heated by a fire, but only gradually, as rapid heating can cause immediate death.[243] Our present explanation for this phenomenon could be from shock; as the circulation improved with the heat, more fluid escapes from the wound area, depleting the blood in the chest and abdominal organs resulting in shock; or death could result from the potassium from the injured muscle entering the restored general circulation, causing cardiac arrest.

> "Never encourage those with slight wounds who are little hurt to stay below, but insist they go back to their quarters, otherwise threaten to report them to their officers after the engagement.

> "I have many times known cowardly lubbers come tumbling down the ladder with most violent groans and complaints, though at the same time they have received little hurt; and all I could do or say would not prevail upon them to take a second trial of their courage, nor go up again till the action was over. Nay, I have been told by those quartered at the same gun that some dastardly fellows have actually put their feet or stood in the way of the carriage on purpose to be hurt...."[244]

After the engagement the surgeon is instructed to give the captain the number of casualties and the prognosis. When the ship is in harbor, the surgeon consults with the hospital surgeon regarding each of the casualties and arranges for the sick and wounded to be brought ashore.

CHAPTER SIX

MILITARY HOSPITALS AND THEIR DIRECTORS

When the war broke out in 1775, Americans had no knowledge and no experience of the direction and needs of a military hospital system. After the establishment of the first hospital at Cambridge, Massachusetts, in July 1775, Washington suggested that as the British had long experience in military matters, that the Americans should organize a system similar to theirs.[245]

As previously mentioned, in wartime, the British established general hospitals directed by a Physician General and a Surgeon General, who jointly appointed the staff. A large convenient building was commandeered for the purpose. Regimental hospitals remained close to the troops and were controlled by the regimental commanders who appointed the medical staff. Field or flying hospitals were established as links between the regimental and general hospital. An Inspector of Pharmacia was in charge of supplies and prepared reports.

After the Battle of Bunker Hill, 350 American casualties were cared for in private homes until June 1775, when the Massachusetts

Provincial Congress established a hospital in Cambridge. Copying the British system of medical support, the Continental Congress in Philadelphia in July 1775 took over the provincial hospital and voted to establish a general hospital for an army of 20,000 men in Cambridge.[246] The Director General and chief physician were to receive four dollars a day, and there were to be four surgeons receiving one and one-third dollars a day, twenty surgeons' mates at two-thirds of a dollar a day, an apothecary receiving one and one-third dollars daily, storekeepers, clerks and one nurse for each ten patients at one-fifteenth of a dollar a day. Such an organization was concerned with a single hospital, not a hospital system.

Regimental and flying hospitals were also to be organized, but not to be under the direction of Congress but provided by the states. Benjamin Church, a prominent Boston physician, was to be the first Director General. The failure of Congress to establish a direct chain of medical command led to divisiveness, rivalries, hostility and bickering. The duties of the Director General were never specifically stated. Was he to control all the general hospitals to be created in the future or just the one in which he was stationed? Was the Director General to provide supplies and command and personnel for the regimental hospitals? The medical staff of the regimental hospitals in Cambridge and throughout the early period of the war expected supplies to be drawn on demand from the general hospital, but refused to accept orders from the Director General and sought to maintain total independence. Congress approved medical appointments to the general hospitals but who was to approve the medical staff of regimental hospitals? The medical committee of the War Board, which was the committee in Congress in charge of medical affairs, failed to appreciate the extended duration of the conflict and its decisions were made on a day-to-day need rather than on the long-term problems arising from battles fought from Quebec in the north to Georgia in the south. The medical committee in Congress had no plan to regularly provide medical supplies, but reacted to sporadic urgent appeals arising from the military situation. Moreover, distribution was chaotic, and pilfering, theft and illegal sale of medical stores was common.

Throughout the war Director Generals, individual surgeons, and field commanders sent urgent pleas to Congress for more supplies, citing wounded soldiers receiving no medical treatment and doctors treating patients without medical supplies. Frequently Congress failed to respond or else provided too little and too late. Congress had meager funds to dispense, and boots, muskets, and munitions had first priority so the purse strings of the treasury were tightly drawn. Reports of medical dissension, doctor incompetence, hoarding of medical supplies, fraudulent reports of hospital census and outright theft of medical items reached Congress and made it very suspicious of medical needs and vouchers.

Congress heard rumors that Shippen as Director General remained distant from the combat areas, living in comfort in Bethlehem or Philadelphia during the battles at Trenton and Princeton and Brandywine and that he maintained excessive personnel where it was not needed. Dr. John Warren at the Cambridge hospital, far from the site of military activity in 1777, was ordered to close his hospital and be reassigned to another general hospital which orders he rejected. Dr. Phillip Turner lobbied to establish a hospital in New London where there was no military activity necessitating a hospital: his motive presumably to draw supplies for personal use. Dr. Isaac Foster, medical director in the northeast department, stockpiled medicine for his own use. To recover these supplies, it was necessary for Washington to send an armed detachment and confront him. Dr. Barnabas Phinney expressed his disgust: "The dirtiest and basest actions are everyday deprecating the profession—till the very appellation (of doctor) had become the butt of satire, ridicule and contempt."[247] Directors of departments, hospital surgeons, regimental surgeons and line officers provided their sponsors in Congress with accusations and tales of perfidy.

American military hospitals throughout the war truly were cesspools of disease where cross infection and contagion were rampant. Some commanders emphasized sanitation and cleanliness, but most were indifferent prompting Benjamin Rush to publish an article in the *Pennsylvania Packet* on April 22, 1777, requesting the medical department to use its authority on line officers to improve the dress, diet, personal hygiene and camp sanitation. Most of the men came from rural areas with no exposure to contagious diseases, which fed on large concentrations of troops. Smallpox, in particular, often decided the outcome of campaigns. In the fighting around Quebec and Montreal in 1776, the effectiveness of the armies of Arnold and Montgomery was destroyed by this disease. Later in the war, Washington insisted that all units be inoculated against smallpox. Military regulations stated that after inoculation of the men, their clothing was to be washed, smoked, and cleansed with vinegar or tar oil; straw bedding was to be burned. In the civilian population, 16% of those infected with smallpox died, but in the military the death rate was higher because of poor nutrition, sanitation and fatigue. Although self-inoculation was severely proscribed, panic-stricken troops frequently resorted to this measure when faced with hordes of their comrades dying.

For every death of a wounded soldier occurring in a hospital, nine hospital patients died of disease. Some of the ills were diagnosed as smallpox, dysentery, putrid fever (camp fever, jail fever, hospital fever), bilious fever (with jaundice), malaria, venereal diseases, rheumatism, pleurisies, nostalgia (indisposition from homesickness).[248]

Many drugs were used and most were of little value, but those that were recognized as efficacious were known as "capital drugs". These were Peruvian bark (quinine) for malaria, elevated temperature and pain; laudanum (opium) for pain, and calomel (mercury) for venereal diseases.

Disease statistics for the British were better, and this might be expected because their soldiers were veterans, better clothed and fed and usually bivouacked in cities and not the countryside. They were enlisted for longer periods and military discipline was more strictly enforced.

Although Americans tried to mimic the British medical department, they succeeded only as far as structuring a similar organization. What they could not include was the long British tradition of operating military hospitals and the duties of the commanding officer in supporting the health of those in his unit. However, the drawing of excess medical supplies caused grumbling in London as well as in Philadelphia. Lord Germaine, the Secretary of War, accused the British doctors of misusing supplies and even suggested that medical items were sold. As in the American forces, friction between hospital surgeons and regimental surgeons existed and was reported to Adair, the Inspector General of the Medical Department in England. The regimental surgeons were supposed to draw supplies from the apothecary except in unusual situations when they could draw them directly from general hospitals. The hospital staff complained of the regimental surgeons and London also thought they were irresponsible in the amount of medicines they drew.[249]

Colonel Anthony Wayne, referring to the American military hospitals during the Revolutionary War, labeled them "houses of carnage."[250] Benjamin Rush called them "sinks, cesspools of human life." At the war's end, Dr. James Tilton wrote in despair of the record of the American army hospitals, stating that the Americans surpassed all other nations in the destruction and havoc committed on their fellow-citizens. Tilton wrote, "It would be shocking to humanity to relate the history of our general hospitals in the early years of the war...when it swallowed up at least one half of our army owing to a fatal tendency in the system to throw all the sick of the army into the general hospital where crowds, infection, and consequent mortality, too affecting to mention..." Amongst the civilian population as well as in the army, a military hospital was regarded with fear and disgust.

Both sickness and casualties were heaviest in the early years of the war. It is estimated that in 1776, 20,000 troops died; one-fifth of all the young eager volunteers joining the army died of sickness, ninety percent of them in a military hospital.[251]

At the time of the retreat of Washington across Manhattan, after his defeat by Cornwallis at the Battle of Long Island, he counted 7,610 men awaiting treatment and only 15,000 fit for duty.

Although more deaths from disease occurred early in the war, the hospital mortality remained high throughout the conflict and little thought or action was taken at any period to reduce this mortality, in spite of the fact that the subject of disease transmission in hospitals had been addressed in European literature repeatedly.

What went wrong? Why did the carnage continue? A number of causes could be explored. The medical directors of the hospital system were treasonous, lacking in tact, personally ambitious and showed mutual distrust and outright rivalries. They were not conversant and familiar with measures to prevent hospital cross-infection. Moreover, they failed to influence line officers of the importance of sanitation.

The Continental Congress failed to understand the enormity of the problem and never organized an efficient chain of command in the medical department. It failed to anticipate the need for supplies, providing them for one emergency after another. Although Congress issued a commission to doctors, it did not offer them rank until the end of the war. Authority in the military can only come from rank. The doctors themselves were not aware of the latest studies in Europe by men such as John Aiken, Sir John Pringle, Brocklesby and others, which placed the blame for hospital epidemics on overcrowding and failure to isolate infectious diseases. Finally, line officers themselves failed to establish their authority in maintaining camp sanitation and discipline within the hospital and policing in the field.

* * * * * *

Benjamin Church, an eminent Boston physician, was appointed first Director General of the hospital in Cambridge. Friction in the medical department was reported to Washington in September, 1775. The regimental surgeons were making demands on the general hospital for supplies which seemed to Church to be far in excess of their needs for bandages, dressings, medicines and equipment. In truth, the regimental surgeons established little empires so well stocked that they were reluctant to send the sick or wounded to the general hospital. Church complained about the expense. Church further antagonized the regimental surgeons by demanding they send all sick patients to the general hospital. The clamor grew, and Washington asked General Greene to investigate. At this juncture, presumably due to the bickering of his fellow medical officers, Church wrote Washington requesting he be relieved of his position. Washington did not accept the letter of resignation, suggesting he was too good an officer to lose. Church, however, had other reasons to leave the military, which gradually came to light.

On September 26, 1775, General Greene requested an urgent interview with Washington. He was accompanied by a baker, Godfrey Wainwright from Newport, Rhode Island. Wainwright was requested to give Washington information he had already related to General Greene. Early in August, a woman approached Wainwright who was situated near the harbor at Providence, and based on a previous acquaintance with him in Boston, asked Wainwright to arrange for a boat to visit a Captain Wallace of *H.M.S. Rose*, anchored in Providence Harbor. Wainwright cleverly discovered the woman had a letter addressed to a Major Cane in Boston and shrewdly insisted that the letter be entrusted to himself for delivery, because of the danger involved. The letter was turned over to Wainwright, who opened it and found a message in code.

The letter was given to Washington and the woman was taken in custody. Wainwright knew her name and indicated she was a woman of easy virtue. Under questioning, she revealed that the letter was given her by Church. Washington and his staff were shocked that the Director General of the medical department, a Boston delegate to the Massachusetts Congress and an avowed patriot, would be sending messages to the enemy. Church was arrested, but some of his papers had already been secretly removed.

On interrogation, Church readily admitted he wrote the letter which he said was intended for his loyalist brother, a book dealer in Boston. Why, he was asked, was it in code and delivered circuitously and in secret? A Reverend Samuel West, who was an expert in secret writing, and Colonel Elisha Porter of the Massachusetts Militia worked independently on the code and submitted identical translations. There was information regarding weaponry, guns and powder which exaggerated the preparedness and strength of the patriots and the letter indicated previous letters had been written.

Washington was convinced the letter was to be ultimately delivered to a high British official, not a book dealer. He laid the matter before a council of his generals and it was decided to hold a court-martial the following day. In his defense, Church said the letter was to discourage British military action. The court found him guilty of treason. This was the first such trial in the military and there was no precedence for action for treason. Treason was not included in the Articles of War by the Continental Congress. Washington referred the matter to Congress, but received no explicit instructions. Church was "utterly expelled" from the Massachusetts Provincial Congress.[252]

For awhile he was set free on his parole, and James Warren wrote, "I fear the people will kill him, if at large. The night before he lodged at Waltham and was saved by the interposition of the selectmen, and by jumping out of a window and flying. His life is of no consequence, but such a step has a tendency to lessen the confidence of the people in the doings of Congress." In 1778, after serving a term in prison, he was released on his bond to leave the country and not return. He sailed on a schooner for the West Indies, but the schooner and its crew never arrived in the West Indies, was never heard of again, and may have been lost in a hurricane. The woman who had been kept by Church was pregnant; Church had disowned his wife. In the Public Record Office in London, there is a statement that a William Warden declared he was sent by General Gage to Salem and Marblehead to receive intelligence from Church.[253] In a later study of General Gage's papers, proof of repeated communications from Dr. Church is presented and showed that he was a paid informant.[254]

Congress on October 17, 1775, appointed John Morgan as successor to Church as medical director of the Continental Army. Morgan received his medical degree in Edinburgh, had toured the medical centers of Europe where he had been introduced to the leading medical authorities. He also had previous military experience, having served with the British in the war against the French and Indians.

When Morgan gave the inaugural address opening the first medical school in America in Philadelphia, William Shippen, M.D., was in the audience and heard Morgan speak of him in a patronizing manner. Shippen never forgot this slight and after Morgan was appointed, leveled charges against him through his friends in Congress. Later, when Shippen became Director General, Morgan's rancor barraged Congress with charges of incompetence and theft of supplies, and lead to Shippen's court-martial. Thus the first and third Director Generals of the medical department were both court-martialed.

When Morgan arrived in Cambridge, he found himself embroiled in the same struggle with the regimental surgeons that had caused Church to request resignation. From the beginning of military action in April, 1775, at Lexington and Concord to the battles around Boston, Colonial militias were the involved military units. Their regimental surgeons fully controlled medical support and directly requisitioned their supplies from their local communities, the Provincial Congress in Boston, and later from the second Continental Congress in Philadelphia.

On July 21, 1775, the Second Continental Congress, at the request of Washington, ordered the establishment of a hospital at Cambridge. Unfortunately, the division of responsibility between those doctors to be appointed by the hospital and those already serving in the militias was not defined. Regimental surgeons were well established in their fiefdoms and regarded the general hospital and Morgan as interlopers. They objected to sending patients known to them from their local

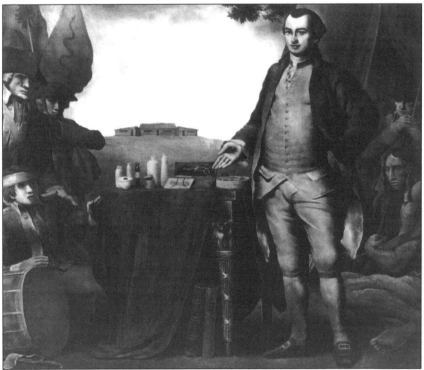

photo courtesy of University of Pennsylvania

John Morgan M.D., Director General of the Medical Department of the Continental Army at Cambridge.

communities to an impersonal hospital. Moreover, the larger the census of patients in the regimental hospitals, the more supplies they could order and thus enhance their power.

Morgan countered by ordering all patients to be admitted to the general hospital and had all supplies sent to the general hospital from which the regimental surgeons must draw them. To make them subordinate, he limited patient rations in the regimental hospitals, threatened to examine the qualifications of the surgeons and requested an inventory of their supplies. Many of the regimental surgeons proved defiant and did not respond. Of thirty-six regiments stationed around Boston, only twenty-four responded and much of what they reported was inaccurate.[255]

These antagonisms continued during and after the Battle of Long Island. Later, they were less acute, but in the absence of any decisive direction from Congress, they simmered throughout the war.

Throughout the early years of the war, Congress was bombarded by letters critical of Morgan. Many of these were from the regimental surgeons, but the most damaging were from Shippen who had many friends in Congress. Congress summarily discharged Morgan on June 9, 1777, giving no reason for his removal. Stringer, Director General in the Northern Department, was also relieved of his duties at this time. Now Morgan, with the aid of Benjamin Rush, started a campaign of his own complaining to Congress about Shippen. Much later Morgan requested a hearing by Congress regarding his discharge as medical director and Congress finally passed a resolution granting him an unblemished record on June 12, 1779. Such divisiveness rendered the medical department even more impotent.

William Shippen, the third medical director, was accused of being an absentee leader. While the battles of Philadelphia and Trenton were fought, he was comfortably billeted in Bethlehem. At the Battle of Brandywine there were no medical plans to treat casualties, of whom there were over four hundred. Many had to be brought almost a hundred miles for hospitalization at Bethlehem after lying in the battlefield for three days.

Morgan and Rush overwhelmed Congress with reports of Shippen's inadequacies and also presented evidence that he was involved in speculation of government supplies for his own profit so that Congress was forced to review the evidence. A court-martial was convened in 1780 in which Shippen was accused of stealing government medical supplies and selling them for personal profit, scandalous practices unbecoming an officer and neglect of duty. In June 1780, the court acquitted Shippen, but in reviewing the proceedings Congress amended the court's findings, accepting the decision of the court on all charges except that part of the second charge relating to his speculating in hospital stores, in which he was judged to be highly reprehensible. He was, however, allowed to continue as medical director.

Morgan and Rush, dismayed at the acquittal, continued to barrage Congress and public opinion with new evidence attacking the integrity of Shippen. One can understand why Morgan persisted and sought the downfall of Shippen. Morgan's good name was impugned by his unexplained dismissal as medical director by Congress which he suspected was due to the conniving of Shippen and his friends.

Rush was Morgan's friend, but the reasons for his zealous efforts to destroy Shippen are difficult to understand. True, he had little respect for him. Perhaps it was the crusading spirit of Rush which he demonstrated in other causes at other times.

Rush wrote to the *Pennsylvania Packet* in Philadelphia in 1780, "A court martial has passed a cold and unanimous sentence by which Dr. Shippen is partially, may I say, dishonorably acquitted." Rush promised the readers that in future issues of the *Packet* he would produce additional evidence to support the charges against Shippen.[256] Rush charged that Madeira wine from the hospital magazine at Lancaster found its way to a local tavern. He also deposed Dr. Tilton, a senior surgeon, who became medical director after the war. Tilton was highly critical of Shippen's decision to divide the large house in Ephrata used for a hospital into monkish-sized cells. Tilton was familiar with the new theory prevalent in Europe which depended on large airy rooms in a hospital with only a few patients in a room to prevent cross infection.

John Hambright, Esquire, was also deposed and criticized Shippen. He also described the hospital at Lancaster. "Its approach and entry was covered with nastiness, its air close and putrid, everything filthy and loathsome; patients cried out they were neglected; wounds hadn't been dressed for days and no adequate nourishment was provided."[257]

Joseph Kimmel of Ephrata was deposed and described sick soldiers arriving on Christmas Day 1777 in open wagons, almost naked, many without shoes and stockings or blankets, without nurses or attendants and left there in the wagons without orders for anyone to receive them. Some of the sick in piteous condition crawled into his and his neighbor's homes where they were treated. His neighbor and wife caught an infection and died treating these unfortunate soldiers. The diseases they carried spread in the community and other benefactors also perished.[258]

The pressure on Shippen was so great that in November 1780 he said he would answer these charges, "...fomented by malicious and wicked people."

In his defense, published in the *Pennsylvania Packet*, Shippen wrote, "I have never denied, for it was unavoidable, that there were many sufferings in the hospitals after the Battle of the Brandywine and Germantown, but the witnesses brought by my enemies proved, when cross examined, that they were not owing to my neglect, to a deficiency of stores or to a want of surgeons, commissaries, nurses, medicines, or other things that I ought or could supply. They arose partially for a want of clothing and the covering necessary to keep the soldiers clean and warm; articles that at that time were not procurable in the country; they were also due partially to the fact that our army was raw and unused to camp life, exposure, fatigue discipline, and great hardships; from their being obliged to flee before an enemy in a cold and inclement season, and under such circumstances the sick and wounded were moved great distances in open waggons. In December 1777, I was ordered by George Washington to remove all the sick from New Jersey and the vicinity of camp into Lancaster County when scarce a waggon was to be had from the quartermaster or flour from a commissary. Notwithstanding all these distressing circumstances, it was effected with little loss and by the uncommon care and attention of the hospital officers. The consequences were not near as fatal as was feared and expected."[259]

Shippen continued as Director General until January, 1781, when he resigned. He had no military or administrative skills and had been ill-prepared for this office. John Cochran, personal physician to Washington, was then appointed Director General and remained in this position until the war's end.

In July, 1776, Congress clarified the role of Director General indicating that he had authority over all hospitals and that there was also to be a director of each general hospital who appointed his own staff.[260] Later, an examination was required for a hospital staff position. A general hospital would be housed in a large building, and regimental hospitals were to be in close support of each regiment whose physicians would be appointed by the regimental commander and supported by the provincial government. In addition to the regimental surgeon, local militias could also enlist the support of a doctor appointed by the community. Drummers and fifers aided by soldiers were employed to drag the wounded from the field of battle where they were then placed on wheelbarrows or wagons and sent to the regimental hospital.

At least one thousand, two hundred doctors served in the military during the war. More American medical officers died in proportion to line officers; evidence that infection is more lethal than the weapons of war.[261] The American troops reporting to training camps were from isolated farms and had little understanding of sanitation and personal hygiene. They were inviting targets for the ravages of communicable diseases that flare up whenever crowds assemble. Moreover, the troops were ill-fed and poorly-housed.

Washington was badly defeated at the Battle of Long Island by Cornwallis who pursued the disease-ridden army across the Hudson River southward through New Jersey. The general hospital at Morristown, New Jersey, housed over one thousand sick and wounded and with Cornwallis approaching, it was thought advisable to establish a hospital at Bethlehem, Pennsylvania. To this peaceful Moravian community the war was somewhere else—a distant struggle not affecting their lives.

On December 3, 1776, Dr. Cornelius Baldwin rode into town to deliver a message from Dr. Warren to the town committee.

"Gentlemen, according to His Excellency, General Washington's orders, the general hospital of the army is removed to Bethlehem, and you will do the greatest act of humanity by immediately providing proper buildings for their reception, the largest and most capacious will be the most convenient. I doubt not, gentlemen, you will act on this as becomes men and Christians. Doctor Baldwin, the gentleman who waits upon you is sent upon the business of providing proper accommodations for the sick, begging therefore that you afford him all possible assistance. I am, gentlemen, your most humble servant, Dr. Warren."[262]

Within a few hours, wagon loads of sick and wounded began to arrive; the men dressed in scant clothing, malnourished and in pitiful condition. The hospital had no supplies and the Moravian community fed and clothed the arrivals and nursed them to the best of their ability. The Reverend Ettwein distinguished himself by his acts of humanity, visiting each of the sick and wounded twice weekly. Ettwein counted sixty-two deaths for December and 110 for the entire occupancy which lasted until March 27, 1777, when the hospital was moved to Philadelphia.

But the Moravians in Bethlehem were soon asked to make even greater sacrifices. With the defeat of the Continental army at the Battle of Brandywine, Philadelphia could no longer be held against the British and in September, 1777, the House of the Single Brethren was again the site of a hospital.

Dr. Shippen sent a letter to Reverend Ettwein in Bethlehem on September 19, 1777.

"My Dear Sir,

"It gives me pain to be obliged by order of Congress to send my sick and wounded to your peaceable village, but so it is. Your larger buildings must be appropriated to their use. We will want room for two-thousand at Bethlehem, Easton, Northampton, etc., and you may expect them Saturday or Sunday. I send Dr. Jackson (Dr. Hall Jackson) before them that you may have time to order your affairs in the best manner. These are dreadful times, consequences of unnatural wars. I am truly concerned for your society and wish sincerely this stroke could be averted, but it's impossible. I beg Mr. Hasse's assistance.

"Love and compliments from my d'r sir.
"Your affectionate and humble servant,
"Wm. D. Shippen, D.G."

Ettwein notes, "On Saturday we began to realize the extent of the panic that had stricken the inhabitants of the capital (Philadelphia) as crowds of civilians as well as men in military life began to enter the town in the character of fugitives."[263]

The House of the Single Brethren quickly was overfilled and tents were put up ringing the hospital with patients arriving from Philadelphia. Generals Lafayette and Woodward were among the wounded. In October, additional convoys of wagons with the sick and wounded arrived, collected from the Brandywine battlefield. Later in October, an additional one hundred patients arrived. The hospital was terribly overcrowded, poorly ventilated and basic sanitation was disrupted. This hospital was regarded as overcrowded when it had 400 patients; there were now 700 sick men in the Brethren's House alone. Doctor Smith of the hospital staff describes how four or five patients died lying on the same infected straw before it was changed; many of those that died were admitted for slight disorders. Upwards of 500 deaths were recorded. Of eleven junior surgeons and mates, ten became infected. Many of the civilian volunteers sickened and some deaths occurred. The army surgeon wished to commandeer the "Sisters' House" and the "Widows' House" but Ettwein strenuously objected and his will prevailed.[264]

Dr. James Tilton had contracted an illness while treating at the hospital in Princeton and on his way home on sick leave stopped briefly at the hospital in Bethlehem. He states, "During my stay it was natural to enquire into the state of the hospital. The method I took was to propose a competition, not whose hospital had done the most good, but whose hospital, the most mischief. I stated well all the exaggeration with truth, not only on affecting mortality among the sick and wounded, but that the orderly men, nurses, and other attendants on the hospital were liable to the infections that I had narrowly escaped and that five other surgeons and mates had afterward been seized. I was answered that the malignancy and mortality of the Princeton hospital bore no comparison with theirs; that at Bethlehem not an orderly or nurse escaped and but few of the surgeons...and to give me some idea of the mortality...that fine volunteer regiment of Virginia commanded by Colonel Gibson.... He then went on to say that forty of that regiment had come to the hospital and then asked me how many I suppose would ever rejoin. I guessed a third of the fourth part. He disclosed solemnly that not three would ever return, one man had rejoined the regiment. The other two were still ill in the hospital."[265]

The day-by-day impact of a large military hospital in a secluded Moravian community far removed from the war and the centers of commerce and politics is graphically shown in the diaries of the Congregation and the Brethren's and Sister's house in Lititz which were translated from the German.[266] The absence of military discipline of the patients is shown in this entry:

"October 21, 1777—During the evening meeting six armed soldiers entered the Sister's House—dreadfully frightening with their brutal swearing, the house watcher and the few sisters who were at home. Their intent was forcibly to enter the dormitory and press for their own use of blankets off the beds. However, they had the goodness to let themselves be dissuaded from their purpose."

"December 14—A Dr. Kennedy brought the news that George Washington ordered that 250 sick and wounded were to be brought to Lititz. Again the Brethren's House used as a hospital. Five days later 80 sick and wounded arrived; 2 days later 100 more;—2 weeks later another wagonload. Both army doctors are ill." The town offered all its services to the hospital. Brother Schmick preached.

(He later died of the fever.) Food was supplied and a graveyard set aside.

"January 10, 1778—Some of our little boys have been trading things with the soldiers, receiving in exchange cartridges and powder which they set off in the barn. Parents were admonished to carefully watch over children and, of course, no one should buy things from the soldiers as it was stolen property."

Another updated entry: "There is no reason why Tobias Hirte should have bought a gun; indeed, on the contrary, it is an unseemliness! What use has a schoolmaster for a gun? He must be ordered to dispose of it."

"March 1, 1778—"Almost 60 well soldiers are rendezvousing here. Their behavior is pretty wild and ill mannered."

Again we have evidence of the lack of discipline in hospitals. Nearly a thousand sick and wounded were quartered at Lititz between December 19, 1777, and August 28, 1778.

The disease problem in hospitals rested squarely on the shoulders of the medical men with some assistance from the Continental Congress which failed to give doctors rank and thus authority. As we have noted, Congress failed to provide adequate food, shelter and medicines. The Director General and physicians spent much of their time fostering antagonisms and charges of incompetence against each other. Issues of control over supplies by the general hospital and whether it was supposed to provide instruments and drugs to regimental hospitals and which patients should remain in regimental hospitals and which patients should be transferred to general hospitals surfaced early in the war and were never fully answered. This polarization and growing embitterment increased suffering and mortality. Even at the close of the war, Congress never clearly established a chain of command; the southern hospitals claiming independence of the Director General.

Medical decisions in the Continental Congress were made by the medical committee of the War Board. At first, three representatives served on this committee. Later, it was expanded to thirteen, of whom seven were doctors. Benjamin Rush served on the committee for a limited time.

At the time Shippen replaced Morgan as Director General of Hospitals, he and John Cochran submitted a plan to reorganize the medical department which was approved by the medical committee and passed by Congress in April, 1777.

Under Shippen's and Cochran's plan the country was to be divided into three medical departments: northern, middle and southern. A physician general who was to be a surgeon was assigned to each district and a Physician General and staff were to accompany the army. Shippen was to be Director General in charge of all departments.[267]

The pay scale was raised and called for the Director General to receive five dollars daily, a senior surgeon four dollars, and a junior surgeon two dollars. By comparison, at this time a colonel of the line received two and a half dollars a day. The Director General was to be an administrator whose function was to establish hospitals, to provide medications, dressings, bedding and furniture, and to submit reports. Assistant directors, apothecaries and a commissary were to be appointed as well as a matron for every one hundred patients and a nurse for each fifteen patients. The surgeons and mates for each hospital were to be appointed by the Director General.

Regimental hospitals were not included in this plan which considered only the Continental army, but Congress did include the flying hospitals, which were field hospitals and were to have a director and a Surgeon General subordinate to the Director General.

The regimental hospitals were usually supported by a doctor from the community. Later in the war, because of the difficulty in getting community doctors to volunteer, the various provincial congresses supplied a doctor and mate for each regiment. Again there was no command structure linking the hospital department and the militias. The reluctance of doctors to volunteer is explained by the fact that a town doctor with a medical degree earned $1,500 annually, a rural doctor about $900, while doctors with the militia earned $20-$25 a month.[268]

This reorganization of the medical department had hardly been put into effect when it was challenged by the hospital in Williamsburg, which declared itself independent of the Director General and the southern department. Congress bowed to this claim and in a separate act declared it an independent hospital. Finally, on February 6, 1778, Congress mustered the resolve that the authority of the Director General be extended to every district.

On March 22, 1777, possibly due to the urging of Benjamin Rush, Congress directed that the commanding general in each division of the army designate separate houses as hospitals so the wounded would be kept apart from the sick. This was never rigorously followed, sometimes because of lack of interest or expedience, or lack of specific communications. In August, 1777, general officers did complain of not receiving congressional resolutions relative to their commands.[269]

Certain principles in the treatment of disease in hospitals had been espoused for many years before the war.[270,271,272] Pringle discusses strict sanitation, rules of personal cleanliness, hygiene of the campsite and avoidance of crowding in military hospitals. Van Swieten also wrote of the diseases incident to armies. John Jones, the American surgeon, in the appendix to his book on surgery, reiterates these concepts; but the pressure of the war, the lack of previous military experience, the indifference of commanding officers, the bickering of the directors and the lack of money and supplies from Congress often caused these postulates to be forgotten and the lessons of previous military hospital experiences in Europe were ignored in this hastily formed army.[273]

Rush suggested that officers must be involved in matters of sickness, wounding and hospitals but again little attention was paid to this suggestion. Rush stated that linen, which was frequently used by the Continentals for shirts, was inferior to flannel. There were to be more vegetables served and less meat; hair was to be cut short, and whole body bathing two or three times a week with fresh changes of clothing were recommended. In encampments, overcrowding was to be avoided, bed hay changed often and placed in the sun whenever possible. Commanding officers were to choose campsites with an eye to a healthy, dry surrounding. Because of lack of interest and money and failure of strict enforcement by the general staff these suggestions were not taken seriously, although they were distributed by Congress to all commanding officers.

The attitude and training of British officers in the total care of troops in their command was compared by Benjamin Rush to that of the Americans. The British officer was described as a father to his troops. The matter of the sick was a matter for the attention of their general officers. Every captain in His Majesty's forces was obliged to visit the sick of his company at least once a day to be certain they were getting full attention. "Considering that sickness sweeps off more men than the sword in all armies, I cannot help but think it is as much a duty of a good officer to save his men by tenderness in the one case as it is...in the other."[275]

In considering the comments on the lack of control of American officers over hospitalized patients and over discipline in general, it should be remembered that Rush was seeking to embarrass Shippen, the Director General, and perhaps even to impugn General Washington. Again, writing on the discipline in the British army, Rush describes an incident when he was treating wounded Americans within the British line at the Battle of Brandywine. On entering the British lines he was challenged by a sentry, marched to the captain of the guard, and then escorted to the wounded Americans. There were strict orders that no British soldier was permitted to touch a dead, sick or wounded American or appropriate his blanket or utensils, lest he contract 'the rebel distemper'.

Within the British lines, Rush discusses a conversation with a British subaltern concerned about his platoon who treats his men like infants, telling them what they can do and what is forbidden. He will not permit his troops to stretch out on the damp grass without a blanket and insists that wet clothes be removed as soon as possible.

When approaching general headquarters on his return to the American lines, Rush was never stopped by a sentry. "I saw soldiers straggling from our lines in every quarter without an officer, exposed to being picked off by the enemy's light horse. I heard of 2,000 men who sneaked off with the baggage of the army to Bethlehem." They would not even be missed because roll call was conducted by a sergeant who made no report to a superior officer.[276]

Rush continues by stating that the waste, theft and the oversupply of unnecessary officers in the medical establishment and the prolonged stay in the hospitals of patients fit for duty would sink the country. This is a political statement directed at Shippen. The system, Rush charges, was formed for the benefit of a Director General and not for the sick and wounded. He further pointed out that many of the hospital inpatients were there for trivial conditions and were drunk each night, often absent without leave from the hospital, and had no assigned officers to supervise their conduct and no sanitary discipline. In Howe's army a captain's guard was assigned for each 200 sick. "We have no guard, and a stay in a hospital undoes all the discipline so carefully instilled into a soldier in his long training."[277]

In the Princeton Hospital many of the 500 sick and wounded had trifling complaints and were at risk of contracting contagious diseases from the sicker patients. Such soldiers should have been cared for in their units, but once in the hospital and under no discipline they were free to commit excesses. The physicians and surgeons, having no rank, had no power to impose order. At Princeton Hospital there were 400 sick and wounded in a house large enough to accommodate only 150, according to the calculations of Sir John Pringle and the American surgeon, John Jones.

On the other hand, the American troops under General von Steuben were trained in the classic Prussian military tradition. Officers demanded strict campsite sanitation and the health of these troops was in contrast to those in other units. The sick were not sent to a hospital but treated in a separate tent in a designated part of the encampment.

In an effort to curb the mounting incidence of venereal disease, which was a problem in this army as in every army previously or since, Congress resolved that the sum of ten dollars be paid by every officer and four dollars by every soldier who entered a hospital to be cured of venereal disease. The forfeited money was to be used to purchase blankets and shirts for sick soldiers in the hospital. The effect of such an order was to deny treatment to those with the disease and to contribute further spreading of the infection.

James Tilton was appointed medical director after the war and in 1781 wrote his book, *Oeconomical Observations on Military Hospitals.*[278] In it he reviewed the many unnecessary deaths in the American forces and laid down rules of conduct to prevent a repetition of such a catastrophe. He studied the measures suggested by Sir John Pringle, head of the British Army Medical Department in Flanders before the American war, and also those of Brocklesby who held that position in the British forces during the war. Tilton also had an opportunity to observe the French military hospital at William and Mary College after the Battle of Yorktown. Pringle and Brocklesby in their writings must be careful not to tread on the toes of the favorites in the monarch's court. In contrast, Tilton recognized his opportunity to speak freely and without reserve in a republican government.

Like Pringle he observed that men were healthier when on the move. Camps became contaminated with filth, excrement, polluted water supplies and fouled bedding straw repeatedly used. He was particularly grieved when reviewing the mortality at the Bethlehem hospital established in the Brethren House. In addition to the mortality of the troops, not an orderly or nurse escaped disease and most surgeons were ill or died.

He noted that the number of hospitals had no bearing on the health of the troops. The French made more hospital beds available than did the British or Germans yet the French lost more men from disease. With more beds than the French, American deaths from disease were highest.

Tilton divided his book into three sections. The first was addressed, "To Ministers of State and Legislatures"; second, "To Commanding Officers"; third, "To the Medical Staff".

In "To Ministers of State and Legislatures", he describes his ideas on organization of the department. The medical director and purveyor of supplies are to be two separate entities with no crossover, so they are a check on each other. At this point he must have been thinking of Shippen who is alleged to have used hospital supplies to enrich himself. All distinction in rank and pay to medical men should not depend on the type of hospital where they are assigned; general, regimental or flying camp. Here he remembers Morgan who made second class surgeons of those assigned to regimental hospitals.

The medical department would be directed by a board composed of the senior surgeon or director and two additional surgeons but the presiding leader of the board is to be a nonmedical field officer. All orders authorized by the board must be sanctioned by the commander in chief. Thus, any officer violating an order would be responsible for his actions to the commander in chief. Tilton details the number of surgeons, nurses, pharmacists per hospital and includes a pay scale.

In part two of his book, Tilton discusses the part played by the commanding officer and all field officers relative to the medical department. He writes, "...that whatever may be the form of government, whether monarchical or republican, the government of the army must be despotic." The commander must adopt a patriarchal attitude toward the army. "General Washington affords a notable example. He was indeed the father of his country as well as the father of the army; and the probity and faithfulness of his character justly entitles him to the appellation. "...happy for America there was in the character of Washington something which enabled him, notwithstanding the discordant material of which his army was composed, to attach both his officer and his soldiers so strongly to his person that no distress could weaken their affection nor impair the respect and veneration in which he was held by them."

From the commander on down, the officers must impose strict health discipline. Clean uniforms, haircutting, exercise, diet are discussed. The digging of privy pits and removal of garbage and carrion for burial are enforced with punishment meted out to offenders. Tents are better than wooden structures as they can be kept cleaner and moved to fresh areas. Earthen floors can be easier cleaned. The plan of construction of a hospital is detailed.

The wounded must be separated from the sick. Only the chronic sick and the wounded were to be treated in large hospitals. Those with acute contagion were to be separated and treated in regimental hospitals.

Part three of the book is addressed to the medical staff. Patients with jail fever, camp fever, dysentery are not sent to a general hospital. Drugs to treat sick conditions are calomel, Peruvian bark and wine. Amputations are to be delayed and avoided, if possible.

Different treatment modalities are discussed, but it is interesting to note that responsibility for disease prevention and sanitation falls to the line officers, not medical men.

* * * * * *

The war in America included major battles with thousands of men pitted against each other, but also firefights in secluded and remote areas between scouting parties and patrols, battles that never were recorded, where casualties were buried in fields and forests and were not reported. The war stretched from Quebec on the St. Lawrence River to the Gulf of Mexico and inland as far as the Mississippi. There is no estimate of those killed in the wilderness skirmishes. This number could equal those killed in major battles. In addition, in battles in local communities between those supporting independence and the Tories, towns and villages were ravaged and feelings ran high so that mass slaughter of men, women and children occurred.

When the British evacuated Boston in 1776, they took with them large numbers of Tories who feared for their lives if left in Boston. These were resettled in Halifax, but throughout the country many remained and fought with the British. At war's end many Tories, whose farms and businesses were confiscated or destroyed and who had lost friends and status, returned to a new life in Britain.

Most major battles went against the Americans. On the other hand, British troop strength was never sufficient to hold an area after it defeated an American force. After the start of hostilities, the British force in America numbered 55,000 men, much too small a number to conquer and hold over a 1000 miles of coastline and several hundred miles westward. In 1777 the British forces were reinforced and numbered 89,000, including 2400 Hessians and an uncounted number of Tories. Later in the war troop strength was reduced to 57,000 as troops were withdrawn to protect the Mediterranean stations and the British

Isles from the French threat in Europe. The average British troop strength throughout the war was 39,196.[279] The militias and the Continental army only occasionally could muster enough men and material to frontally oppose a large British force. Washington's strategy was to fight a guerilla type of war attacking small military posts, supply lines, and rear guard actions. In his favor was the knowledge that the British could not commit enough troops to hold their gains because of their European obligations and the staggering financial drain necessary to support an army 3000 miles across the Atlantic. If he could keep his small army viable and win sufficient victories to maintain the enthusiasm for independence, success could be a reality.

The greatest number of Americans died of disease in camp and in hospitals. That number in the Continental army is given as 8,128, but this does not include statistics from the local militia nor does it include Americans dying in British prison camps or prison ships; nor does it include Americans discharged from hospitals or their units as absent sick, who returned home and then died.

About 5,000 Americans were captured after the Battle of Long Island. To the British these men were not prisoners of war, but rebels, mutineers, treasonous to the king, and were thus herded into vermin-infested houses or imprisoned in old ship hulks rotting on the Hudson River. They were given meager rations, no clothing, allowed no fires to protect them from the cold winter, and provided no medical care. Smallpox and "putrid fever" took their toll and one-half of them did not survive, dying in wretched circumstances; an inglorious end to their patriotic response to the call of liberty and freedom. *The New Hampshire Gazette* of April 26, 1777, wrote, "The enemy in New York continues to treat American prisoners with great barbarity. Their allowance to each man for three days is one pound of beef, three worm-eaten biscuits and a quart of salt water. The meat, they are obliged to eat raw, as they have not the smallest allowance of fire." The paper reported that in the short period of three weeks, 1700 prisoners died. They had been herded in a tightly confined space with meager rations and minimal treatment.[280] The number may be exaggerated but others have attested to the barbaric conditions of the New York military prisons. A Lieutenant Collins narrated that he and 225 other American prisoners were loaded on board the British ship *Glasgow* on December 25, 1777, crowded between decks, bound for Connecticut. Eleven days later when the ship made port, 28 bodies were removed.

The best known of the many prison ships anchored in the Hudson River was the *Jersey*. Anchored on the Hudson River, her masts and rigging removed, she held more than 1000 American prisoners, herded into her worm-infested hull and guarded by brutal Hessian soldiers. There was no medical aid, no heat throughout the winter months; dysentery and typhus took their daily toll. Each night the guards battened down the hatches; each morning, on opening the hatches they called out, "Rebels, turn out your dead."

James Fox, a prisoner held on board the *Jersey*, wrote, "I now find myself in a loathsome prison among a collection of the most wretched and disgusting looking objects that I ever beheld in a human form. Here was a motley crew covered with rags and filth, visages pallid with disease, emaciated with hunger and anxiety and retaining hardly a trace of their original appearance."[281]

The dead bodies, unceremoniously thrown overboard, washed up on the Long Island shore with each ebb tide. The *Jersey* and other prison ships rode at anchor throughout the war in Newport, Halifax and Charleston.

The British refuted American claims that treatment aboard prison ships was barbarous, with inadequate food, crowding, no sanitation and no medical care. After the denial there was a terse admission of the American claim by a Dr. Jackson of the British army: "...there was no help for it, it must be done."[282]

After the Battle of Yorktown, it was the British who complained about American treatment of prisoners. The terms of surrender included providing treatment for the wounded, but after the victory they were left unattended and forced to fend for themselves. Of the more than 6,000 troops who surrendered, 1,545 were in the hospital, many of whom were forced to wander around the countryside seeking whatever help they could find.[283]

The total number of Americans killed in action is best estimated to be 7,174.[284] A much larger number died of disease. Most of the smallpox deaths were between 1775-1777. In the latter years of the war most of the army was inoculated. Two hundred and fifty thousand Americans fought during the six years of the war which was 9% of the population.

Duncan estimated that sickness in the American forces was 200 per year, per thousand men; the British sickness rate was 100 per year, per thousand and the Hessians suffered 62.5 per year, per thousand.[285] The last figure is the most reliable as the Hessians, under their medical director Dr. Schoepf, kept accurate records.

In regard to battle deaths, Duncan estimates the Americans lost 20 per thousand men, per year, with an average strength in the field of 40,000. And if the length of the war is estimated at six years, the total figure is 4,800.

The British battle deaths were estimated at 18 per thousand, per year and the Hessians at 18-75 per thousand, per year.

The number of wounded relative to killed varied according to the tactics of individual battle developments, but in general two or three were wounded for each soldier killed. At Bunker Hill, the American dead were 140. In the rout of the Americans at the Battle of Brandywine in Pennsylvania, 300 were killed, 300 wounded and 315 captured. Most casualties in the southern campaign were sustained at Camden, South Carolina, in 1780 where 250 were killed and 300 wounded.

In another report, those killed in action in the army and navy are listed by name. Between the years 1775-1783, a figure of 9,500 is given.[286] The best estimate of death from disease from this source is 18,500.

Jefferson, in a propaganda statement made to encourage the French to aid the American cause, stated that 8,800 British were killed prior to 1777. A British Whig journal, which was critical of the Tories in power in London, stated that 8,848 Britons had been killed, 9,875 injured and 10,161 captured in the Colonial War.

In review, the most accurate figure is difficult to arrive at, but the best estimate would be 25,500 Americans killed in action or died in service of which 18,500 died of disease and 7,000 died in action.

Chapter Seven

CIVILIAN HOSPITALS

T he first hospitals in Europe were an outgrowth of almshouses where the paupers and homeless were given shelter and treated by physicians who volunteered their services. A person of means would under no circumstances consider admission to such an institution. Later, these hospitals were divided into an almshouse for care of the needy indigent, and what we know today as a hospital where ill patients were treated.

In the early eighteenth century, Paris was the medical center of Europe. It boasted of the leading physicians and medical authors, including Jean Louis Petit, Pierre Dionis, Pierre DeSault, Jean Pierre David, Nicholas Andry and Francois LeDran. Ambroise Paré, the military surgeon, published numerous books on war surgery as early as 1545, and his influence continued to make Paris the center of medical advances.

Later, the Edinburgh School of physicians instituted bedside teaching and de-emphasized the use of Greek and Latin in their instruction. This school also subscribed to the experimental method which had been applied to medicine by John Hunter and thus, gradually, the center of medical thought shifted to Britain.

By the eighteenth century, hospitals devoted themselves exclusively to the care of the destitute-sick and were described as houses of horror, condemning inmates to death. John Aikin, in 1771, described his thoughts on hospitals: "The physician...when he walks through the long wards of a crowded hospital and purveys the languid countenances of the patients, when he feels the peculiarly noisome effluvia, so unfriendly to every vigorous principle of life.... He will look back upon a hospital as a dismal place where the sick are shut up from the rest of mankind to perish by mutual contagion."[287] Patients infected their fellow patients until the entire hospital was rampant with disease. Hospital fever was the name ascribed to the most common disease. "That dreadful distemper, little less malignant than the plague itself, distinguished by the title of the jail or hospital fever has long been know as the inbred pestilence of crowded receptacles for the sick and has thinned out fleets and armies, more than the sword or the enemy. Even in a good uncrowded hospital, a slow depressing fever creeps over the patients' other complaints and becomes the principal disorder."[288] Mostly this condition was typhus, but in reality it must have been a group of infectious diseases including dysentery, a variety of enteric conditions, as well as other diseases most of which could and did lead to a prompt death.

Although Aikin had no concept of a bacterium or a virus, he recognized that some agent spread disease when people were crowded together. He wrote, "...that every person by his breath and the effluvia arising from his body vitiates the air."[289]

John Jones, the American surgeon, has an appendix in his book on hospitals,[290] and noted that in the small country infirmaries in England, the death toll of the hospital population was much lower than in the large London hospitals of St. Bartholomew or Saint Thomas, and the death rate from the same disease in those patients treated in their homes was even lower than the country infirmaries. Jones described hospitals as pesthouses. In the large London hospitals 600 people died each year of hospital incurred disease, about one in thirteen admissions. In the small Northampton infirmary, one of nineteen admissions died.[291]

After Jones received his medical degree, he continued his studies throughout Europe. At the Hôtel Dieu in Paris, which was a prototype of the large city hospitals later built in the nineteenth century in America, 22,000 patients were admitted each year of whom one-fifth died. Jones described the appalling conditions in this hospital on making morning rounds. "It is impossible for a man of any humanity to walk through the long wards of this crowded hospital without a mixture of horror and commiseration at the sad spectacle of misery. Beds in triple rows with four to six patients in a bed. In making rounds in the morning, I have found the dead lying with the living. The number of patients overwhelms treatment."[292]

The means to overcome this tragic situation was known to those doctors in the forefront of medicine, but were not employed until much later in the following century. Jones attributed the spread of disease to overcrowding and poorly constructed hospitals. He recommended structures be built with good ventilation, large airy rooms with no more than eight patients in a room. Soiled dressings must be quickly removed and burned and the floors sprinkled with vinegar. Aikin was even more specific. There must be less crowding and beds were to be aired daily. The hospital must be constructed as a series of rooms opening into a wide airy gallery to prevent the spread of disease, but also, "...to avoid the shocking view of the patients from their neighbors dying in hideous agony."[293]

The reduction in the number of patients in a room, and the emphasis on large airy, well-ventilated rooms is in line with the prevailing concept of the eighteenth century, that disease arises by inhaling foul air or air exhaled by a sick patient. Control of temperature, air changes, and humidity therefore were necessary for a healthful environment and prevention of disease which under crowded conditions spread from one person to another.

Aikin emphasized that not every patient who is ill is to be sent to a hospital. A selection is to be made. Contagious diseases and cancer patients are not to be sent to a hospital. The former, because of fear of spreading the disease; the latter, because being in the hospital could not lead to a cure of the disease. Fractures and injuries should be admitted to a special hospital and large cities should have accident centers. In the United States, Aikin's recommendation for trauma centers evolved two hundred years later.

Scrofula (draining tuberculosis abscesses) should not be admitted because of the "misery of the patient and because the hospital can't cure the condition." On the other hand, venereal diseases should be admitted because it was thought that victims could be treated successfully with mercury compounds. If smallpox patients require hospitalization, they should be admitted to a special hospital for this problem and he recommended that inoculation for this disease be vigorously pursued. Aikin added, "There is not in the whole annals of the healing art any discovery so beneficial to mankind as is the practice of inoculation." (Smallpox vaccination as distinct from inoculation was not yet a reality.) Aikin also noted that hospitals serve a purpose for teaching students and cited Edinburgh as the best example.[294]

Patients admitted to hospitals who were injured or mildly ill frequently contracted lethal diseases from their fellow patients. John Pringle in England, Benjamin Rush, and others commented and wrote about this problem; those physicians concerned attributed the hospital spread of disease to overcrowding and inhalation of the toxic air from sick people contaminating the new admissions. Hospital construction was a topic discussed by many leading physicians at this time. Wards were to contain few patients and should be constructed so they surround a central building. Ceilings were to be high and air vents were to be built between the walls and roof. A large fire in the central control room created a draft that circulated air and smoke through the vents. The smoke itself was thought to be a purifying agent and the burning of tarred rope or wood was often employed to detoxify the air in the presence of disease.[295]

Pringle, serving as a military surgeon with the British forces in Northern France, noted that sick soldiers sent to the hospital showed a new set of symptoms after arrival and unexpectedly died; all of the hospital patients exhibited the same symptoms prior to death. If, because of improper orders, absence of transportation, or any other reason that prevented an equally sick soldier from reaching the hospital, the disease ran its course, no new symptoms developed and the soldier quickly returned to duty.[296]

Philadelphia, the most populous city in the colonies with a long history of freedom of thought and religious tolerances, assumed medical leadership in America and the first hospital, the Pennsylvania Hospital, was built in 1751, long before the opening of the medical school. We have no record of overcrowding or a high death rate of admissions to this hospital which was closely associated with Dr. Thomas Bond, its leading physician. Bond, educated in the Edinburgh tradition, instituted bedside teaching in this hospital soon after the medical school was established. Bond was also impressed with Morgagni's book, *Seats and Causes of Diseases*, and Bond used this hospital to lecture the students on the importance of the autopsy in making a correct diagnosis and learning about disease. Morgagni, in Padua, Italy, carefully autopsied patients whose clinical condition and symptoms were known and recorded before death, and he related the findings at postmortem to the clinical course of the patient.[297] Although Bond used this hospital to instruct medical students of the importance of autopsies, there is no record that Bond published any studies in this area.[298]

The New York Hospital was the second hospital built in America and was designed by John Jones, professor of Surgery at Kings' College. Jones, with his personal experience of the miserable conditions in European hospitals, was also familiar with the recommendations for hospital construction made by Pringle, Aikin and others which he quotes in the appendix of his textbook on surgery. Here was his opportunity to put theory into practice and design an airy, well-ventilated structure with no more than eight patients in a ward.

The hospital received a charter in 1771 and was constructed as planned, but before it admitted its first patient it burned in 1775. When partially rebuilt, it was requisitioned for American troops who occupied the building, until the defeat of Washington and his army at the Battle of Long Island in 1776 when the American forces were driven from the city, and it was then occupied by the British who remained until the end of the war.

After the war, the hospital lay vacant for several years, and in 1788 it provided the opening scene in the drama of the New York mob riots. Permission had been granted to Dr. Richard Bayley to use one of the rooms for dissection and student teaching. An account of what happened is best described by William D. Duer, president of Columbia College, in his *Reminiscences*.[299]

"On Sunday, the 13th inst. (1788) a number of boys, we are informed, who were playing in the rear of the hospital perceived a limb which was imprudently hung out of a window to dry; ...a multitude soon collected...entered the hospital; and in their fury destroyed a number of anatomical specimens...several young doctors narrowly escaped the fury of the people; and would inevitably have suffered very seriously had not his honor the Mayor, the Sheriff and some other persons interfered and rescued them by lodging them in gaol.

"On Monday the crowd demanded to visit and inspect the homes of the physicians involved and did so. Later in the afternoon a mob formed and demanded the doctors to be turned over to them; the mob persisted and the militia were called to suppress the riot—one contingent went through the crowd unmolested, but a second contingent of 12 militia were attacked and their arms seized. The mob tried to break into the gaol, but were resisted by those militia still in service. The mob was reinforced in the evening and a heavy barrage of stones and brickbats were used against the defenders with some injured. The militia then fired, and three or four persons were killed and the mob dispersed."

In 1791 the hospital reopened and was used for teaching by the medical school of Columbia College, later the College of Physicians and Surgeons. No other hospitals were chartered during the Colonial regime although military and temporary hospitals were established.

CHAPTER EIGHT

RESEARCH, NEW IDEAS

P hysicians and surgeons were well educated, and although looked upon by the common people with some suspicion, were well accepted in the society of intellectuals. Benjamin Rush described a dinner he attended given by Sir Joshua Reynolds, and meeting the renowned Samuel Johnson, the American painter Benjamin West, and the author and playwright, Goldsmith.[300] Physicians were the majority members of the Royal Society and published treatises in the field of natural history, including botany, astronomy, geology, and chemistry as well as medicine,[301] and to enter medical school they had to pass courses in these subjects. It is not surprising that the leading naturalists of this era were physicians such as Haller and Linnaeus.

With such an elevated status, their opinions were often sought in politics, and they assumed a leadership role in their communities. The premier American scientific group in the Colonial period was the American Philosophical Society in Philadelphia with many physicians as members; its prime mover was Benjamin Franklin who wrote articles on medical subjects, and the society included as members John Bartram, botanist, Thomas Bond, physician, Samuel Rhodes, mechanician, William Parsons, geographer, and Phineas Bond, natural philosopher. In its *Transactions* in 1771, there were articles on medicine, mathematics, and natural history. In one issue of the *Transactions*, Franklin described the use of a bellows to provide air for a drowned person, an improvement on mouth-to-mouth resuscitation.[302]

The resuscitation of persons drowned or with other acute problems was addressed by John Fothergill who described an Humane Society in England to treat apparently dead persons after an acute episode. The society awarded two guineas to any person attempting such a rescue and four guineas if successful. Fothergill reported the treatment of a person suffocated by fumes in a burning coal mine who was apparently dead, while a doctor blew air into his mouth and revived him in front of an audience of several hundred people.[303] Fothergill recommends such treatment after lightning, self-inflicted hanging, and strokes.[304]

Humane societies were formed in Boston and Philadelphia, and treated drowned, hypothermic and other individuals by warming the body, pinching the nose and blowing into the mouth to elevate the chest; tobacco smoke was also blown into the rectum through a lighted pipe with the stem in the rectum. Many case histories of success were recorded at their meetings. Hanging the person upside down or rolling over a barrel, the usual remedies for these conditions were regarded as ineffective.

American doctors continued playing a leading role in public life. In the early days of the republic the number of medical men who were legislators, governors or occupied position of public trust in the developing government was surprisingly large. Five of the fifty-six signers of the Declaration of Independence were doctors as were twenty-three members of the Provincial Congress of Massachusetts in the trying days of 1774-5. Physicians in the government included: Arthur Lee, Minister to France in 1776; Sam Holton, President of

Humane Society

OF THE

Commonwealth of MASSACHUSETTS:

WITH THE

RULES

AND

For regulating faid SOCIETY,

The Methods of Treatment to be ufed with Perfons apparently dead; with a Number of recent Cafes proving the happy Effects thereof.

BOSTON: Printed in the Year 1788.

Summary of the Method of Treatment to be ufed with Perfons apparently dead from drowning.

CONVEY the perfon to the neareft convenient houfe, with his head raifed;—Strip and dry him as quick as poffible; clean the mouth and noftrils from froth or mud—if a child, let him be placed between two perfons naked, in a hot bed—if an adult, lay him on a hot blanket or bed, and in cold weather, near a fire—in warm weather, the air fhould be freely admitted into the room.—The body is next to be gently rubbed with warm woollen cloths fprinkled with fpirits, if at hand, otherwife dry;—A heated warming-pan may be now lightly moved over the back, properly covered with a blanket—and the body, if of a child, is to be gently fhook every few minutes:—Whilft thefe means are ufing, one or two affiftants, are to be employed in blowing up tobacco fmoke, into the fundament, with the inftrument provided for the purpofe, or a Tobacco-Pipe, if that cannot be had—the bowl filled with Tobacco, and properly lighted, being covered with a handkerchief, or piece of linen, fo as to defend the mouth of the affiftant in blowing; Bathe the breaft with hot rum, and perfift in the ufe of thefe means for feveral hours. If no figns of life

Humane societies provided emergency treatment. Anyone attempting resuscitation received an award of money from the society, which was doubled if the person survived. Mouth to mouth breathing or the use of a bellows in the mouth was also recommended.

Congress in 1780; James McHenry, Secretary of War under Washington, and many others.

In America more than in Europe, physicians attempting to study anatomy or the clinical problem in medicine and surgery were obstructed by religious and cultural restrictions placed on human dissection and study. In Philadelphia, William Shippen, professor of anatomy at the College of Philadelphia, had his house attacked by an angry mob, convinced he was robbing graves to procure anatomical specimens. As we have already noted, riotous mobs in New York City, convinced that doctors were robbing graves for anatomical material, viciously attacked them.[305]

* * * * * *

Students were taught that a single form of treatment was applicable to all diseases. Modifying Galen's theory, groups of physicians adhered to one theory or another, arguing the merits of their concepts. Physicians were encouraged to think in terms of systems of disease and unity of treatment. Most doctors considered that all disease had a common cause and treatment. The eighteenth century was the setting for an explosion of information in the physical sciences. Astronomy could predict the eclipses of the sun and moon, the paths of comets, and the orderly arrangements of the planets and their satellites; the mathematics of gravity first promulgated by Newton established unifying principles and was shown to be applicable to a wide diversity of problems in the physical sciences. Doctors were fascinated by the simplicity of such unity and reckoned that in medicine, too, underlying general principles governing disease remained to be unearthed. Its discovery was vigorously pursued in armchair metaphysical reflections.

Such thinking meant that a specific diagnosis was unimportant as a common treatment would be applied to all conditions, and that even measles and smallpox, both of which could be individually diagnosed by blemishes on the skin or crusts, required the same treatment. A few exceptions where specific treatment was recommended did occur. In the case of venereal disease, mercury was relied upon and when applied to syphilis it was partially effective. Rush, in America, strongly recommended the usual therapy for yellow fever but specifically insisted on the additon of mercury, which was of no value. The bark of the cinchona tree from South America, which contains quinine, was recommended for all febrile diseases, where it was effective in reducing the fever, and particularly effective when the fever was due to malaria. Laudanum, a product of opium, was effective in reducing pain. Few other remedies were of any value.

The medical unifiers in the eighteenth century continued to follow the precepts of Galen, that there was no one specific disease but that all illness arose from an imbalance of the body fluids, and that symptoms exhibited by the patient were an attempt to throw off the offending fluids. Fever and sweating removed fluids through the skin. Emetics and purgatives caused vomiting and diarrhea, which also was beneficial, and the doctor could also remove impure blood by bleeding the patient. An enormous number of drugs, usually extracts of herbs or mineral substances, were relied upon to correct the imbalance and many of these were poisons if given in sufficient dosage. They included arsenic, mercury, antimony, lead and others. To increase removal of fluids from the skin, plasters of irritating material and cupping were used. The theory of toxic air as a cause of disease was gradually supplanting the humoral theory at this time but treatment remained unaltered.

How did the illness develop within the person? It could develop from within as a failure of physiological processes, but increasingly, in this century it was felt to be an external toxin, and most often, it was thought to be from impure air. Most theories of disease transmission blamed polluted air. Pollution could arise from an ill patient exhaling air or from smallpox crusts on the skin or other body particles blown into the atmosphere; or it could arise from humid, stale, excessively cold or warm air descending on a community. In certain seasons of the year the air might be contaminated with a specific disease; yellow fever was expected in the late summer air, sore throats in the winter air. The exhalations of many people crowded together on a boat, in a jail, or in a hospital, triggered disease. Foul air entering a wound resulted in gangrene or mortification of an extremity.

If air is the responsible agent, then a study of the weather might throw some light on the origin of disease. Studies of this kind were frequent and John Lining in Charlestown, South Carolina, published such a study in the *Transactions of the Royal Society* in 1744. Lining continued an in-depth report on himself for a full year, recording his pulse frequently and weighing himself twice a day, calculating his fluid intake and output and his state of well-being in relation to air temperature, wind force, air humidity and whether it was raining, cloudy or sunny. No conclusions were reached.[306]

William Heberden in London undertook a most ambitious epidemiological study to determine the number of mortal diseases reported between 1701 to 1790 in London. His figures were taken from the "weekly bills of mortality" (death certificates), and, unfortunately, he had only six broad categories of diagnoses with which to work—deaths from childbed, consumption, fever, colic or flux, measles or smallpox.

He sought to determine if patterns of mortal diseases depended on the environment or occurred in cycles and whether they were rising or diminishing. Heberden realized this was a difficult study as many deaths were unreported and the diagnosis even within these broad categories was poorly made. Nevertheless, he concluded that throughout the century the death rate and the causes of death in London remained unchanged.[307]

In New York, James Hardie recorded meteorological observations in relation to a yellow fever epidemic. He minutely pinpointed the areas where the first victims were recognized near the wharves of the waterfront. A person reported a ship recently arrived from Hispaniola had the foul water of her bilge pumped into the harbor near the wharf just before the first case was diagnosed. From this location on the waterfront, Hardie located the houses of people acquiring the disease and related the rapid spread to high temperatures and heavy rainfall, "the venom" being exhaled from the sodden ground, rising into the air and fouling it. He contributed an excellent epidemiological report showing areas of the city where new cases were concentrated, but failed to associate the spread of the disease to any vector but the air.[308]

Hardie discusses the question of where the disease arose: locally, or was it imported, and favored the former idea, but many in the city thought it was imported, and, later, laws regarding quarantine of ships were passed.

Noah Webster, although not a physician, was deeply interested in philosophical inquiry and wrote several books on medical subjects. After the yellow fever epidemic in New York in 1795, Webster published a collection of articles by various physicians trying to unravel the enigma of the epidemic in New York, sometimes called remittent or bilious fever, but better known as yellow fever. Dr. Valentine Seaman ascribed the epidemic to heavy rainfall and damp weather and remarked that the "...musquitoes were never before known by the oldest inhabitants to have been so numerous."

The epicenter of the epidemic was near the low ground and docks of the city; in this limited area 500 people died of the disease in three months. Filth and stagnation also were rampant in this area. Seaman concluded that the "toxic effluvia" arose from the mudflats and correctly concluded the disease not to be contagious. He told of farmers from outside the city who brought their produce to city markets and manifested the disorder in their local community on their return distant from the city, but the disease did not spread to their families and neighbors. He concluded from this that it was not contagious. He suggested that the rotting docks be torn down, low areas filled in, and an improvement made in sanitation.[309]

John Hunter, as a military surgeon assigned to Jamaica in the mid-eighteenth century, also wrestled with this problem and was more interested in cause rather than the treatment of yellow fever. He kept careful notes of the disease and published a book of his experiences.[310] Some British regiments sent to the island lost fifty percent of their personnel in a single year from the disease. On the other hand he notes that American regiments sent to Jamaica fared much better with a lower mortality partly because they were inured to the disease on the American continent, but also "because they were more orderly and less guilty of drinking to excess." Hunter noted that crews who remained on board in the harbor rarely suffered the disease, but the men in their water details assigned to fill the water casks on land contracted the disease. Shore troops assigned to lowland areas had much more disease than those stationed at higher altitudes. "The air on the land is pernicious and is particularly poisonous in swampy areas." Hunter wrote numerous letters to the war department in London requesting they change the stations to a higher altitude, shrewdly alluding to the economic savings that could be made if troops didn't have to be constantly replaced. He was much affected by the misery and suffering of his troops but thought the economic argument would get a better response. He was wrong; no change was ever made.

Hunter was also able to sort out two disease entities from his studies in Jamaica. Remittent fever with its high death rate and yellow skin and eyes was yellow fever. Intermittent fever with its more benign course and its regular recurrence was probably malaria.

Smallpox and measles, which were clearly and definitively diagnosed by skin changes, were properly considered to be spread from a diseased person. Some enlightened individuals considered passage of all disease to be transmitted from individual to individual not the air.

John Hunter spoke about a "virus" that could be responsible for disease,[311] but the concept could not be tested. The air as a source of disease fit comfortably into a single theory which explained all disease. There was no reason, therefore, to alter the usual individual treatment.

Pringle in England delivered an address on air and its functions to the Royal Society on November 30, 1773, on the occasion of a medal to be presented to Joseph Priestley, discoverer of oxygen.[312] Pringle was one of the most respected physicians in this period. His *Observations on the Diseases of Armies*,[313], in which he described disease transmission in hospitals was widely read and referred to by John Jones, Benjamin Rush and others in America.

Pringle acknowledged the work of Priestley on oxygen and Boyle on his discovery of the relation between volume, pressure and temperature of gases, and showed a profound understanding of barometric pressure, the weight of air, its ability to transmit sound and its necessity in support of vegetable and animal life. Some air is toxic and causes disease: air in mines, or over fermenting material, was artificial or factitious and could not support the flame of a candle. Air is injured by the breath of an animal or by the burning of fuel. Health, therefore, was dependent on pure air and disease from befouled air.

Quarantine as public policy was reported as early as the seventeenth century. In 1689, smallpox again appeared and ravaged New York City, and one of the first statutes of quarantine is noted. The Common Council of the City of New York decreed that

> "William Lynes, Master of ye ship 'Anne and Catherina', arriving here from Nevis with a parcell of negroes where and some have ye small pocks Ordered that all which are sound in Body may be landed, cleaning themselves sufficiently, and those which are sick to be Landed a mile or thereabouts from the City and to Permit none to come to

them but ye doctors, Chirurgeons and attendors."[314]

The council thus recognized that contact with the ill was dangerous and that keeping them at a distance was also important. Quarantine of ships carrying infected passengers and crews was increasingly ordered, as multiple epidemics took their toll on the city, and Bedloe's Island, the present site of the Statue of Liberty, was assigned as a quarantine station and known as the Pest House.[315]

When yellow fever appeared in New England in 1647, John Winthrop noted,

> "...a great epidemic with a high mortality exists in the Barbados and the suspicion arose that the disease was imported by a vessel from the Barbados.... The report of this coming to us by a vessel which came from Fayal, the court published an order that all vessels which came from the West Indies should stay at the Castle and not come on shore, nor put any goods on shore without a license on pain of 100 £ fine."

In 1663 New Amsterdam (New York) was experiencing a severe smallpox epidemic and in an effort to prevent its spread to Connecticut, the Connecticut General Assembly issued an order.

> "The Court, understanding that the hand of God is gone against the people in New Netherlands by pestilential infections, do therefore prohibit all persons from any of these places into the Colony."[316]

Individuals, houses, or neighborhoods would be isolated. In severe epidemics, many people left their homes and sought refuge, distant from the infected area.

* * * * * *

A few doctors broke with the tradition of rationalism and sought specific agents that caused a specific disease. An impetus to such a radical view was the discovery in Europe that scabies was associated with the mite, *acarus*, which could be seen with a magnifying lens. Cases of scabies were seen to be associated with the mite. No one went so far as to try to transfer the mite to a healthy subject to see if the disease could be passed this way, but if mercury was applied to the skin, the mite disappeared as well as the itch. The physician Giovan Cosimo Bonoma and the apothecary Giacenta Cestoni in the late seventeenth century discovered this pathogen. If this disease can be transferred from person to person by an animaliculum, why not others? Van Leeuwenhoek had seen many tiny animals swimming in a drop of water under his microscope lens—could not these, too, be related to disease?

The doctrine of contagium vivum received further verification from two physicians in Padua. In 1711 a plague developed among oxen in Venice. The outbreak was traced to a single ox shipped from Hungary. Antonio Vallisnieri and Carlo Francesco Cogressi put a drop of the infected ox's blood under a crude microscope and saw tiny worms crawling in the drop of blood.

> "A living thing rather than an inanimate thing, can pass from man or animal to another man or animal and it can multiply."

Vallisnieri also suspected that time was necessary to produce sufficient worms until the whole composition of the blood "...is thrown into confusion..." We now term this an incubation period.

Vallisnieri also wrote,

"...that even this pestilential race of tiny little vermin was established by God in the creation of the world for His own lofty purposes, that they are always alive in some body, that perhaps their native land is beyond the mountains and the seas, and that even there, they do not always display their ferocious nature, either because they are hidden away in some niche or not always so fierce or are few in number...they wiggle from place to place as an invisible army."

The investigator is wrestling with new concepts, finding a place in the organization of biology for a new species of life, and he must explain how they arrived in Venice, where they came from, why they did not always produce disease and how they spread. He touches upon ideas used in our time of toxic dose, endemic conditions, alterations in pathogenicity and virulence and transmission.

Cogressi goes further adding that,

"...to subdue a living agent of disease, it would suffice to find one remedy alone...perhaps one growing in the garden of the poor."

These worms can be lifted into the air on a piece of straw or grass and transported. If an amulet is worn containing mercury or some other substance, it may protect the individual and chase away the worms.[317]

The oxen contagion was severe and widespread and no cure was found, but a new idea was born which was immediately attacked and satirized. One must consider the possibility that the "worms" swimming in the blood seen by Vallisnieri and Cogressi were contaminants which entered the blood after it was removed from the ox blood which is a good culture medium for parasites. The worms could thus play no part in the cause of the disease of oxen. Whether this is true of not, full credit must be given the investigators for a new concept. The courage to depart from conventional thinking was the leap of the mind to a new plane.

Consumption, phthisis or tuberculosis was prevalent in England and America, and with no clue to its cause, its treatment was relegated to one of the many diseases that are explained by a theory. Galen regarded this condition as being caused by a peculiar malignant and corroding humor from inhaling toxic air.

Benjamin Marten of London had heard of the animaliculae seen floating about under the lens of a microscope. From his experience, he knew the disease was frequently seen in families and, in his book, postulated that a certain species of these animaliculae, breathed in the air from exhalations of one individual, were deposited in the lungs of another to cause the disease. Marten was familiar with the writings of Nicholas Andry in Paris who wrote, "...if we considered the infinite number of these little animals which microscopes discover to us...and that a great quantity of them may enter the Body of Man...where they are then brought to life...and by their growth...may cause diseases besides what we treat of..."[318]

Marten also theorized that other diseases could be caused by different organisms, the ova of which were breathed in the lung. One such animal "...may offend the brain and nerves, others could cause apoplexy, plague, scurvy, gout, rheumatism, leprosy, and other diseases."

As expected, Marten's brilliant insight was denounced and severely criticized. His detractors leered when he was asked to describe his treatment, which was the same as those of other physicians. Marten and Andry were among those first to show a glimmer of understanding leading to the germ theory of disease.[319]

The power of the microscope was so limited that further study of this idea had to wait over a century before the tubercle bacillus could be demonstrated. The definition of Van Leeuwenhoek's microscope was adequate to describe and trace the life history of fleas. He even described a mite that attacked a flea, which prompted Jonathan Swift (1667-1745) to write:

> So, naturalists, observe a flea
> Has smaller fleas that on him prey,
> And these have smaller still to bite 'em
> And so proceed ad infinitum.[320]

* * * * * *

Thomas Jefferson, who was critical of theories of disease, and the medical establishment noted how physics, chemistry and astronomy were making great forward strides while medicine was stalled in this century. In a letter to Caspar Wistar requesting him to look after his grandson, Mr. Randolph, who was going to Philadelphia to study medicine, he suggested that courses in anatomy, chemistry and natural history should be encouraged, but he withheld approval of courses in medicine. "It is in this part of medicine, I wish to see a reform, an abandonment of hypotheses for sober facts." Referring to the young medical student, "...his mind must be strong indeed, if rising above juvenile credulity, it can maintain a wise infidelity against the authority of his instructors and the bewitching delusions of their theories."[321,322] Jefferson's opinion of doctors is revealed in his statement, "...that whenever he saw three physicians together, he looked up to see whether there was not a turkey buzzard in the neighborhood."

The average doctor was frequently the butt of jokes by others than Jefferson. As far back as the seventeenth century Samuel Purchas, a parson in Ludgate, England, said a physician is like a fly, "Always visiting sores and ulcers..." they often kill instead of curing. He tells of a woman concerned about the future of her sons, "...that woman which

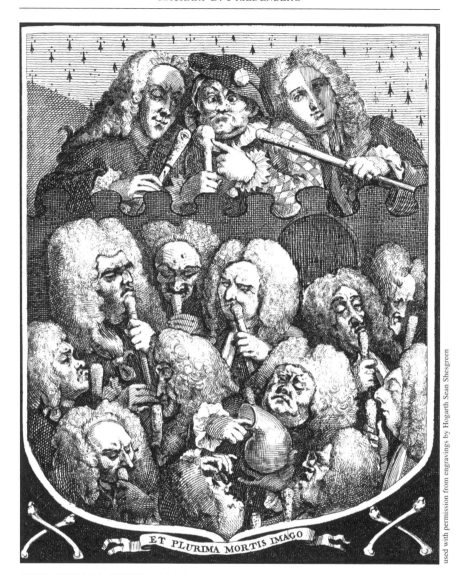

ET PLURIMA MORTIS IMAGO (and many an image of death).
Lack of respect and mockery of the medical profession. This coat of arms for the medical profession is a satirical representation of the profession. The doctor pointing to the bone is a bone setter. Doctors sniff the disinfectants on the canes and dip their fingers into the urinal.

much dreading her three sonnes, one to incurre the law for his meddling; the second likely to produce a murtherer by his bloudy frayes;

the third by unthrifty courses like to become a beggarie, was advised to make the first a lawyer, the second a physician, the third a divine...."[323]

The principal cause of death and suffering in this century was infection which often swept across communities as epidemics exacting a frightening toll. Throngs of city people fled into the country at such times, intuitively recognizing that disease spread by proximity of one individual to another and that the disease having settled in an area would wreak great calamity. Without knowledge of bacteria or viruses and no certain knowledge of the cause or spread of the epidemic, the physician remained at his post treating the sick to the best of his ability while exposing himself to the disease daily and frequently becoming a victim. Benjamin Rush describes the heroism of the doctors in Philadelphia during the yellow fever epidemic in 1793, remaining in the city to treat patients while all those who could do so fled the city.[324]

Theories of disease had been postulated in the seventeenth and in the eighteenth centuries by Sydenham, Boerhaave, Cullen and others in Europe and by Rush in America. Common to all these theories was that external matter deranged the interior balance of the body but nothing specific had ever been identified and the manner of spread of this external matter was unknown.[325] As we have seen, occasionally physicians sought other explanations of disease, not being content with holistic theories. The spread of epidemics and transmission of disease to families and neighbors suggested something other than foul air, something specific which must be passed from victim to victim. Certainly this was known to be true in smallpox. Francis Home of Edinburgh was sure a specific factor must be transmitted in measles, a diagnosis which is easily made, with a death rate at that time of 8%. He took blood from measles patients and transferred it into the veins of recipients seeking to introduce the disease. He tried it on thirteen cases and was not successful in passing the disease.

Home followed Hunter's advice to Jenner, "Don't think, try...." Unfortunately, he was unsuccessful.[326]

To Pringle in London we owe not only a quest for this information but also a method of proceeding, utilizing a modern scientific protocol with controls. Pringle had studied with Boerhaave and Van Swieten in Leyden and later practiced in Edinburgh, following which he was a physician in the British army. In his book, *Observations on the Diseases of the Army*, first published in 1752, there is an appendix entitled, "Experiments Upon Septic and Antiseptic Substances".[327]

This series of experiments involved placing human serum in vials with other substances such as muscle to determine if putrefaction or decay developed, which he recognized by clouding of the vial, loss of integrity of the putrefying substance and odor.

Substances that retarded putrefaction were "antiseptic", those that increased putrefaction "septic". Urine, when added to the vial, delayed putrefaction compared to a control without it. The vials were placed in the sun or near a furnace and the temperatures in some instances recorded.

Alkalis (spirit of Hartshorn) were antiseptic and delayed putrefaction of muscle when kept one month in the summer. Salts of tartar or wormwood as acids also were antiseptic but a mixture of acid and alkali failed to delay putrefaction. Myrrh in water was twelve times more antiseptic than seawater. Sixty grams of salt was a better antiseptic than thirty grams. Pringle then proceeded to rate various salts in the same concentration as to their effectiveness.

And then came an experiment which surely must have ignited his imagination. A thread was dipped into a vial with a putrefying egg yolk, and a piece of the soaked thread presumably carrying bacteria placed in a vial with fresh egg yolk. The vial with the thread putrefied the experimental egg yolk faster than a control with no thread. Experiment XLII involved placing the blood of an ill person into a vial and heating it. The control vial continued clear four times longer than

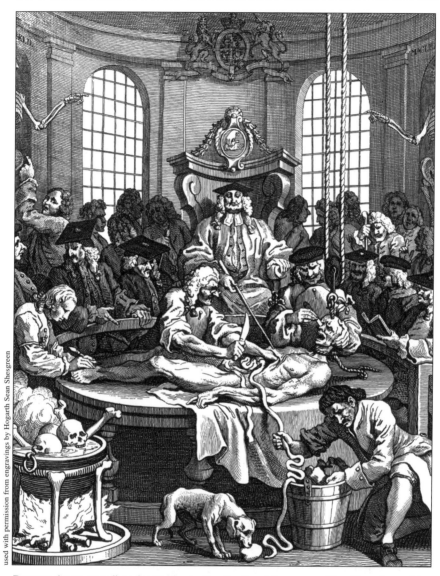

Doctors shown as sadists, insensitive to the dignity of the corpse. Tom Nero, hanged by the state with the rope still around his neck, is given over to the doctors for dissection. In this engraving by Hogarth in 1751, the shield of the Royal College indicates the site of the anatomy lesson, above which is the Royal Coat of Arms. The doctor in the center conducts the lesson, but the attending doctors pay little attention, reading, joking and conversing while the dog feeds on the heart.

the experimental. He communicated his results to the Royal Society in 1752 in a series of articles titled, "Experiments Upon Septic and Antiseptic Substances with Remarks Upon Their Use in Medicine". Pringle was poised on the brink of a major discovery, yet he was so bound by tradition that he continued to believe that air, not some specific substance in the air or his vials, was the cause of the putrefaction or fermentation. Pasteur over 100 years later identified bacteria as the cause of tissue destruction.

In America references to Pringle's book were made by John Jones and Dr. James Tilton of the Continental army as well as in the textbook of surgery by Nicholas B. Waters published in America.[328,329,330]

Rush introduced Pringle's book to his medical students in America, praising the book, but cautioned them not to take it too seriously, particularly the part about antiseptics, for Pringle's experiments, he said, do not apply to a living body. Rush continued to teach that all disease is airborne and arose from a single cause, morbid excitement, and that no other ideas are to be entertained about disease or its treatment.[331]

William Alexander in Edinburgh refers to Pringle's book on putrefaction and continued similar experiments, but failed to use controls. He used entire animals, seeking to prevent putrefaction by soaking the exterior but was blind to the fact that the circulation of the animal also must be made antiseptic.[332] He soaked his own feet in an antiseptic substance (Peruvian bark) and then noted his urine was antiseptic, again with no control study.

Medical quackery, masquerading as scientific advances, presented theories which quickly gained public support. In Europe, Mesmer's theory of animal magnetism had swept the Continent. When Lafayette returned to America after the war, he tried to convince his friends of the force inherent in electromagnetism and its therapeutic value. Jefferson regarded Lafayette as a fanatic, and most Americans had a healthy mistrust of Mesmer's ideas. However, Dr. Elisha Perkins devised a set of "tractors" or short metal rods which were magnetized and used to point out the seat of disease and to cure it.

Elisha Perkins (born 1741) was apprenticed to his physician father after he graduated from Yale. He noted that a live muscle touched with a metallic instrument contracted, which he presumed to prove Mesmer's ideas about animal magnetism. He formed two strips of different metal three inches in length and pointed at one end which could attract and draw out disease if passed over the affected part of the body. Perkins sold large numbers of his tractors with his trademark stamped on the metal for five guineas. The tractor craze soon swept over Europe, a Perkinean institute was founded in London, books were published, free treatment was provided to the indigent, and the Royal Academy of Copenhagen sponsored a book which was translated into English and German. Miraculous cures were described and successful treatment reported even on horses.

A debunking experiment was done in New York in which patients who were blind and lame recovered after "Perkins Tractors" were passed over their affected areas. When told Perkins Tractors were not used but were substituted by kitchen skewers, symptoms returned. The author describes how mankind is consistently deceived by the same tricks played over and over again. Why is medicine singled out "as the playing field for deception? What man would have his tailor shoe his horse or his barber build his boat?"[333] Benjamin Douglas Perkins defended his father and presented him as a persecuted individual, comparing his trials to those of Galileo and Copernicus, and prophesized that in the future his discoveries would occupy a place of honor next to those of Volta and Galvani.[334] In America there was little enthusiasm for the method and the tractors' ability to cure was completely discredited.

Thacher in his autobiography stated,[335] "Such is the history of the metallic tractors. It is to be considered a singular and unaccountable circumstance that the remedy should be consigned to oblivion. Is it within the bounds of probability that the vast amount of authenticated evidence that has been produced should be resolved into a delusion, a mere phantom of the imagination?" Today, such a question could still be asked of the many remedies that appear on the scene, only to be soon forgotten.

While foreign nations were adulating Perkins, he was expelled form the Wyndham County Medical Society in 1797 because of his patents and unscientific conduct.

* * * * * *

In medicine, for the most part, little progress was made during the eighteenth century. Theories of medical practice prevailed and the individual maladies were lumped into a confused mass with little knowledge emerging about their specific characteristics, course, and treatment. The one outstanding exception was smallpox which was well described and its course known. Prevention of this disease by inoculation was almost universally accepted by the end of the century. Vaccination for smallpox in the last years of the eighteenth century prevented the scourge of epidemics of this disease that had terrified the world for centuries. Venereal diseases were treated with mercury which was partially effective for syphilis. Laudanum and quinine were effective drugs. Most other drugs had no effect on the course of illness.

As the century closed, Morgagni in Italy and others emphasized the importance of autopsies, and the pathology of various diseases slowly began to be understood. Some leaders in medicine were showing that diseases were seen to affect different organs and in different ways.

In America, four medical schools were graduating well-educated doctors. Some restrictive legislation in the various states limited those who could practice on the public, as licensure was increasingly required. Hospitals were established and medical journals were published.

In the century to follow the trickle of understanding of disease symptoms and pathology, and the role of a single organism as the cause of disease by medical leaders in the nineteenth century became a torrent which unravelled the complexities of most diseases; but effective treatment would not be forthcoming until the twentieth century.

* * * * * *

In surgery, as in medicine, research methodology for proving or rejecting a concept was still far in the future, but the alert minds of people seeking answers kept grappling with problems. The vagaries of both man and his culture sometimes offered strange opportunities for scientific advancement.

Maggi, an army surgeon in Italy and later professor at Bologna in 1542, published a book seeking improvements in reconstruction after amputations by observing the wound healing problems of thieves who were punished by amputations at the wrist by the lictors of Venice. Recognizing the need to resurface the wound, he covered the wound with a graft using the skin of a freshly killed fowl and published his conclusions and ideas on skin grafting in 1542.[336] Ambroise Paré published books on the treatment of gunshot wounds in 1545 and later, and probably gained some of his ideas for the treatment of wounds from Maggi.[337]

John Hunter in London also wrote about gunshot wounds. He was one of those rare people that never accepted the approved explanation of an event, but must test it and provide his own answers, whether in the field of comparative anatomy, biology, medicine or surgery. He fired the minds of his students, many of whom were Americans, and stirred them to rebel against long held sacred theories.

In this era most surgeons advocated and practiced extending a wound, enlarging it so foreign matter and bone fragments could be removed, and to control bleeding. Hunter strongly opposed this wound extension except in certain instances where severe hemorrhage must be controlled by ligating an artery. He also acknowledged the necessity of wound extension in the case of head injuries associated with a fracture to reduce the pressure on the brain of displaced skull fragments or when abdominal organs are eviscerated.[338]

Benjamin Gooch, a British surgeon from Norwich, disagreed with Hunter and described an eight-year-old boy who died because his wound was not extended. The boy fractured his leg and had a pinpoint opening over the fracture site. Gooch was asked to consult because the condition of the child was rapidly deteriorating. He described the entire limb and lower abdomen as being emphysematous, infiltrated with gas. Gooch made incisions into the swollen tissues and described the hissing sound as gas escaped from the wound. The boy died two days later with gas-filled tissue rapidly advancing to the navel. Gooch claimed that the child could have been saved if the surgeon had extended the wound soon after it occurred. This was an obvious case of gas gangrene and a radical enlargement of the wound was necessary to prevent development of this complication and to allow air to enter the anaerobic gas-filled tissue. The possibility that the child could have been saved by these measures applied early is in accord with present medical knowledge.[339]

Hunter, on the other hand, illustrated his theory of not enlarging wounds with an experience in his brief career as a military surgeon in Spain. Four men wounded in the extremities took refuge in a shed during the battle without any treatment for four days. When they were found by Hunter, they were all doing well with wounds beginning to heal. Hunter was convinced that interfering with the natural process of wound healing led to a poor result.

As a military surgeon, Hunter's interest turned to the effects of musket balls in tissue. He set up an experiment noting the effect of the ball on cadavers. A low velocity ball caused little damage, making a path through the tissues and failing to fracture the bone; higher velocities caused increased tissue damage and splintered the bone; while still higher velocities resulted in severe tissue damage and drilled a neat hole in the bone, rather than shattering it.

In ballistic studies 200 years later the additional damage done by high velocity bullets was fully appreciated. Such a bullet entering the tissue creates a wave of increased pressure in the course of its track and the pressure itself creates a cone of destruction. Hunter's study of firearms led to his remarks about firearms which seem true today. He noted, "...and it is curious to observe that firearms and spirits are the first of our refinements that are adopted by uncivilized countries."[340,341]

Hunter set out to study how bone grew. Was it interstitial growth, the whole bone taking part in the elongation, like stretching a rubber band, or did it grow from a specific region? He drilled two holes a measured distance apart in the middle of a bone of an immature animal and placed shot in the holes. The marked holes did not change their distance apart with growth of the animal, proving that the bone grew from a specific area. Later, he fed madder, a red dye, to growing pigs and showed that the dye accumulated mostly at the ends of the bone in areas that had grown since the animal fed on the madder. He also showed that some dye accumulated under the covering of the bone or periosteum and that later this surface dye was transposed to the inner surface of the bone. Hunter failed to determine the significance of this very interesting phenomenon but his observations were accurate. With aging the exterior shape of the bone was being remodeled and some of the original dye deposited on the surface of the shaft was now on the interior of the shaft as it increased its diameter.[342]

He also performed complicated and dramatic experiments in tissue transplantation. A "Christian's tooth" survived in a cock's comb as did a chick's testicle in a hen.

Hunter correctly identified the stages of a healing fracture noting that the gap is originally a cavity filled with hemorrhage which later is vascularized and is replaced with cartilage and bone. The surgeon's role is "to bring the ends of the bones together and it then heals." The failure of a fracture to heal is still a problem today and usually overcome by metal fixation and bone grafting. Hunter recommended opening the refractory fracture and exposing the ends to permit increased tissue to form in the gap, even allowing the bone ends to rub on each other and increase the inflammation by not completely immobilizing it. The concept of allowing micromovement rather than rigid immobilization is recognized today as advantageous in forming a strong bond or callus uniting the bone ends.

Duhamel, in mid-eighteenth century France, also discussed the healing of fractures. It is not certain that he did any research but he concluded that the covering of the bone like the bark of a tree acts to heal a fracture assisted by structures from within the cavity of the bone. Haller and his pupil, Dethleef, performed experiments in animals and mistakenly concluded that a jelly-like fluid exuded from the bone ends united a fracture.[343]

LeDran, in France, conducted studies of gunshot wounds to learn about their distant systemic effects which he divided into stages of commotion, syncope, coldness and convulsions. It would seem that such effects would result from hemorrhage and shock due to wounding rather than the gunshot wound itself. Like Hunter, he fired pistol balls into a cadaver from varying distances to study the damage done.

Studying his injured patients, he showed unusual perception in describing a condition known today as "compartment syndrome". He demonstrated that a membrane covering a muscle also dips into and surrounds the muscle or groups of muscles as a sheath. Inflammation (swelling) strangles the muscle within the sheath. "The forearm swells, becomes hard and a gangrene ensues. Incisions should be deep and unbridle all the parts,...chiefly the tendinous membranes." The part may have to be removed if release does not work.[344] In

America, John Jones' instructional book on military surgery draws heavily on LeDran's book.

Philip Syng Physick, professor of surgery at the University of Pennsylvania, sought the proper material to suture a wound. Like so many other American medical students, he had studied with Hunter after his graduation from Edinburgh and was imbued with Hunter's quest for new knowledge.[345]

Physick also described the use of a stomach tube used on two children, twins, who came under his care after an accidental dose of laudanum given by the mother for convulsions to treat an attack of whooping cough. Physick examined them and noted they were lethargic with depressed respirations and feeble pulses. In London, he had seen Hunter pass a stomach tube made of eelskin. He then passed a flexible catheter, possibly made of gum rubber, into the stomach of Edmund and instilled some ipecac, an emetic, down the tube with no effect. He then attached a pewter syringe and applied suction, repeatedly instilling water and withdrawing it, pumping the stomach, still without effect. The patient appeared dead, so he injected some spirits and vinegar into the tube, following which the child started to breathe. The same treatment was given his brother, William. The next morning William was dead, but Edmund survived.[346]

* * * * * *

As the eighteenth century closed, progress in surgery had been made and disseminated. Wounds from injuries were to be enlarged and allowed to fill in; when mature they could be closed. Bleeding was controlled and ligation of blood vessels was widely practiced. Musket balls and splinters were removed from wounds, if accessible. More attention was to be focused on the direction and velocity of a ball, and wounds of entrance and exit distinguished. Improved instrumentation was designed, such as musket ball and arrow extractors, spoons, borers, trephines and forceps. Ideas about what wounds required amputation and the timing of amputations were beginning to crystallize.

Most surgery in this century was concerned with amputations and the treatment of wounds. A few elective procedures such as removal of bladder stones, cataracts, superficial deformities, as well as repair of herniae were performed. Surgery was limited to simple operations which could be rapidly completed to limit the pain suffered by the patient. It was also necessary that no incision into a body cavity remain exposed to the air for lengthy periods to prevent contamination from the "toxic air". Complex surgery was impossible under these conditions.

The stage was set for a tide of new advances in the following century which would provide the means to practice detailed surgical procedures. In the nineteenth century, bacteria and viruses as the cause of infection and the development and understanding of anesthesia provided the springboard for the leap of surgery in the twentieth century.

GLOSSARY

Animalculae   Living moving organisms seen under the micro-scope and regarded in the eighteenth century as miniature animals.

Asepsis   A procedure in which all instruments, drapes and equipment, as well as the skin are sterilized for an operation.

Axilla   Under the arm.

Body humors   Four fluids which must be in balance to preserve health. According to the physician Galen, these are black bile, yellow bile, blood and phlegm.

Commotion   In the eighteenth century, a bodily disturbance such as inflammation.

Disarticulate   To amputate a limb through a joint.

Febrile disease   Any disease associated with a fever.

Fistula	Abnormal connection between two organs or between an organ and the skin in which fluid flows.
Fomentation	Treatment by warm, moist dressings.
Occlusive dressive	A dressing that completely covers a wound.
Pulsatile	A rhythmical pulsation.
Sacral sores	Skin openings adjacent to the pelvic sacrum.
Scarify	To create a scar.
Scorbutic	Related to scurvy — a Vitamin C deficiency.
Scrofula	An Abscess caused by tuberculosis.
Septicemia	An infection of the blood stream usually by a bacteria spreading throughout the circulation.
Stricture	Decrease in the caliber of a vessel or duct as a result of scarring or abnormal growth of tissue.
Suppuration	The formation and discharge of pus.
Syncope	Fainting, swooning.
Tenaculum	An instrument with teeth to grab and hold tissue.

Trepanation
  (Trephination)

Removal of a circular disc of bone usually in the skull to gain access to the brain.

Variolous matter

Pus or crusts from a smallpox sore.

Viscosity

Thickness of a fluid which impairs its rate of flow.

REFERENCES

1 Bush, V., *Endless Horizons*, Public Affairs Press, Washington, D.C., 1968.

2 *The Dreadful Visitation of the Plague on London in 1665*. Defoe, Daniel. Republished by Henry Miller, 2nd Street, Philadelphia, 1767.

3 DeBonneville, G., *Medicina Pennsylvania*, handwritten text circa 1770.

4 Packard, F. J., *Practice of Medicine in the New England Colonies*, Journal American Medical Association, May 7, 1898.

5 Blake, J. B., *Public Health on the Town of Boston*, Cambridge Press, 1959.

6 Wesley, J., *Primitive Physick*, Robert Hawkes, London, 1772.

7 Blake, J. B., *Public Health on the Town of Boston*, Cambridge Press, 1959.

8 *From God's Controversy with New England*, Massachusetts Historical Society, Proc. XII, 7871-3, 1991-2.

9 Butterfield, L. H., *Letters of Benjamin Rush*, Vol. I, Princeton University Press, Princeton, New Jersey, 1951.

10 Radbill, S. X., *The Barber Surgeons Among the Early Dutch and Swedes*. Bulletin Inst. of History of Medicine, Vol. VI, December, 1936: from Der Arzt und die Heilkunst in dei deutsche vergangenheit, H. Peters, Leipzig 1900, p.78. Translated by Samuel X. Radbill. From an original in 1568.

11 Keith, A., *In Contributions to Medicine and Biology Research*, p. 549, Paul Hoeber, New York, 1919.

12 Jones, J., Plain Concise, *Practical Remarks on Treatment of Wounds*

and Fractures. Robert Bell, Philadelphia, 1776.

13 Blanton, W. B., *Medicine in Virginia in the Eighteenth Century.* Garrett and Massie, Richmond, Virginia, 1931.

14 Floyer, J., The Physician Pulse Watch, Printed by S. Smith and B. Walford, St. Paul's Churchyard, London, 1707.

15 Shryock, R. H., Germ Theory in Medicine Prior to 1870. Clio Medica V7, 81-109, Amsterdam, 1972.

16 Buchan, W., *Advice to the Populace.* Cruikshank, London, 1774.

17 Blanton, W. B., *Medicine in Virginia in the Eighteenth Century,* Garret and Massie, Richmond, Virginia, 1931.

18 Whipple, A. O., *Evolution of Surgery in the United States.* Thomas, C. W., Illinois, 1963.

19 Beck, J. B., *Medicine in the American Colonies,* Horn and Lovelace, Albuquerque, New Mexico, 1966.

20 Rush, B., *Lectures on the Practice of Physick.* Manuscript, University of Pennsylvania Library 1, no. 31 and II no. 1, 1796.

21 Radbill, S. X., Thomas Jefferson and Medical Education. Address to Thomas Jefferson Medical College, December 3, 1969.

22 Thomas, O., From a letter to Caspar Wistar, Mayo Clinic Procedure, V47, March 1972.

23 Pringle, J., *Observation on the Diseases of the Army.* Published by Royal Society, London, 1752.

24 Pringle, J., *Observations on the Diseases of the Army.* Published by Royal Society, London, 1752.

25 Pringle, J., *Diseases of the Army.* First American Edition with Notes by B. Rush, Edward Earle, Philadelphia, 1810.

26 De LaCondamine, M., *The History of the Inoculation of Smallpox,* T. S. Green Publisher, New Haven, Connecticut, 1773.

27 Shryock, R. H., Letter to Woodward quoted by George L. Kittredge, Massachusetts Historical Society, Proc. XLV 422, 1954.

28 Anonymous. The Abuses and Scandals of Some Later Pamphlets in Favor of Inoculation by A.S.M.D. printed by J. Franklin, Boston, 1722.

29 Thacher, J., *American Medical Biography,* Printed by Richardson and Lord, 1828.

30 Anon, Letter to Zabdiel Boylston, Occasioned by a late Dissertation concerning Inoculation, printed by D. Henchman, Boston, 1733.

31 Waring, J. J., *A History of Medicine in South Carolina; 1670-1825*. Published by South Carolina Medical Association, 1964.

32 Thacher, J., *Modern Medicine*. Ezra Head, Boston, 1817.

33 Gibson, J., Dr. Bodo Otto, Charles C. Thomas, Baltimore, 1937.

34 De LaCondamine, M., *The History of the Inoculation of Smallpox*, T. S. Green Publisher, New Haven, Connecticut, 1773.

35 Jenner, E., *On The Origin of the Vaccine Inoculations*, printed by N. Shury, London, England, 1901.

36 Jenner, E., *On The Origin of the Vaccine Inoculations*, printed by N. Shury, London, England, 1901.

37 Jenner, E., *Varieties and Modifications of the Vaccine Pustule*, printed by H. Ruff, Cheltenham, England, 1806.

38 Jenner E., *An Inquiry into the Causes and Effects of the Variolae Diseases*, printed by D. N. Shury, London, England, 1801.

39 Lettsom, J., *Observations on the Cow Pock*, printed by Nichols and Son, London, England, 1801.

40 Aikin, C., *A Concise View of All The Most Important Facts Concerning Cow-Pock*, (2nd American Ed) printed for J. Groff, Philadelphia, Pennsylvania, 1801.

41 Waterhouse, B., *A Prospect of Extermination of the Small Pox*, printed by W. Hilliard, Boston, Massachusetts, 1800.

42 Lettsom, J. *Observations on the Cow Pock*, printed by Nichols and Son, London, England, 1801.

43 Ibid.

44 Lettsom, J. *Observations on the Cow Pock*, printed by Nichols and Son, London, England, 1801.

45 Waring, J.J., *A History of Medicine in South Carolina*, 1670-1925. Published by South Carolina Medical Association, 1964.

46 Chisholm, W. C., Description of the American Yellow Fever, in a letter by John Lining, Thomas Dobson, Philadelphia, 1799.

47 Waring, J. J., *A History of Medicine in South Carolina 1690-1925*, Published by South Carolina Medical Association, 1964.

48 Lining, J., *Statistical Experiments, Philosophical Transactions*, Woodward and Davis, London, 1744.

49 *Gazette of the United States and Advertiser*, July 30, 1794, printed and sold by Thomas Dobson, Philadelphia.

50 Middleton, Wm. S., *The Yellow Fever Epidemic in Philadelphia of 1793*, Annals of Medical History, 10, pp.434-450, 1928.

51 Butterfield, L. H., *Letters of Benjamin Rush*, Vol I (1761-92), Princeton University Press, Princeton, New Jersey, 1951.

52 Packard, F.R., *Practice of Medicine in New England Colonies*, Journal American Medical Association, May 7, 1898.

53 Hunter, J., *Treatise on the Venereal Disease* (American Edition), Printed by Parry Hall, Philadelphia, 1791.

54 Ibid.

55 Hamilton, R., *Dissertation on the Marsh Remittent Fever*, Printed by J. Newman in the Poultry, 1801, London.

56 Hamilton, R., *Dissertation on the Marsh Remittent Fever*, Printed by J. Newman in the Poultry, 1801, London.

57 Waring, J. J., A History of Medicine in South Carolina; 1670-1825. Published by South Carolina Medical Association, 1964.

58 Buchan, W., *Advice to the Populace*. Cruikshank, London, 1774.

59 Elliot, J., *Complete Collection of the Medical and Philosophical Works of John Fothergill*, Printed by John Walker, London, 1781.

60 Caulfield, E., *The Throat Distemper*, which occurred in His Majesty's New England Colonies between years 1735-40. From Disease and Society in Provincial Massachusetts, Arno Press and New York Times, 1972.

61 Bard, S., *Enquiry into the Nature and Cause of Angina Suffocativa*, Printed by Inslee and Car, Beaver Street, New York, 1771.

62 Elliot, J., *A Complete Collection of the Medical and Philosophical Works of John Fothergill*, Printed by John Walker, London, 1781.

63 DeBonneville, G., *Medicine in Pennsylvania*, Hand Written Manuscript, circa 1776.

64 Elliot, J., *A Complete Collection of the Medical and Philosophical Works of John Fothergill*, Printed by John Walker, London, 1781.

65 Heberden, W., *Commentaries on the History and Cure of Diseases*, New York Academy of Medicine, Hafner Publishing Company, New York, 1962.

66 Editorial, *The Science of Medicine.* Medical Journal and Record V125, 198-201, 1927.

67 Jackson, J., *Memoir of the Last Sickness of General Washington.* Privately printed, Boston, 1860.

68 Solis-Cohen, *S., Washington's Death and the Doctors*, Privately Printed, Philadelphia, 1940.

69 Archer, J., *An Inaugural Dissertation for the Degree of Doctor of Medicine* to Rev. John Ewing, provost, and the Trustees and Faculty of the University of Pennsylvania, 22 May 1798.

70 Blanton, W. B., *Medicine in Virginia in the 18th Century*, Garrett and Massie, Richmond, 1931.

71 Jackson, J., *Memoirs of the Last Sickness of General Washington.* Privately printed, Boston, 1860.

72 MacLehose, J., *The Observations of Hawkins, R., Knight, in His Voyage into the South Sea.* Samuel Pruchas, Editor, Hakluytus Posthumus, or Purchas His Pilgrims, 17, Glasgow, Scotland, 1966.

73 Aikin, J., *A Specimen of the Medical Biography of Great Britain*, printed by J. Johnson, St. Paul's Church, London, 1775.

74 Ramson, D., *Review of the Improvements of Medicine in the 18th Century*, Printed by W. P. Young, Charleston, S.C., 1800.

75 Lind, J., *An Essay on The Most Effectual Means of Preserving the Health of Seamen.* Printed by D. Wilson and G. Nichol in the Strand, London, 1774.

76 Beddoes, T., *Observations on the Nature and Causes of Calculus and Sea Scurvy*, printed by T. Dobson, South Second Street, Philadelphia, 1797.

77 Trotter, T., *Observations on the Scurvy*, Elliot and Robertson, London, 1786.

78 Van Swieten, G., The Diseases Incident to Armies, Translated by Raney, J., American Edition, published by R. Bell, Third Street, Philadelphia, 1776.

79 Bell, W., *The Clinical Notebook of John Archer*, MD.., 1768.

80 Bell, W., *An Eighteenth Century American Medical Manuscript.* The Clinical Notebook of John Archer, MD.., 1768.

81 Dorsey, J., *Daybook*, 1806.

82 Thacher, James, *A Military Journal During the Revolutionary War*, Printed by Cotton & Barnard, Boston, 1828.

83 Waters, Nicholas B., *System of Surgery*, (extracted from the Writings of Benjamin Bell,) T. Dobson, Philadelphia, Pennsylvania, 1791.

84 Earle, A Scott, *Surgery in America.* W. B. Saunders, Philadelphia and London, 1965.

85 Wangensteen, Owen H.; Smith, J.; Wangensteen, S.D., *Some Highlights on the History of Amputations.* Bulletin History Medicine XLI, 1967.

86 Gooch, Benjamin, *Chirurgical Works*, Printed by J. Johnson, London, 1792.

87 Dorsey, J.S., *Elements of Surgery*, published by Parker, E. and R., and Benjamin Warner, Philadelphia, 1818.

88 Abernathy, J., *Surgical Observations on Injuries of the Head*, Printed by T. Dobson, Philadelphia, 1811.

89 Blake, J., *Diseases and Medical Practice in Colonial America*, Int. Rec. of Medicine v. 171, 1958.

90 Buchan, W., *Domestic Medicine*, Printed by John Cruikshank, 1774.

91 Freke, J., *An Essay on the Art of Healing*, Printed by W. Innys, 1748.

92 Butler, J. R., *Lectures in Surgery* by Philip S. Physick and J. J. Dorsey, Hand Written Notebook, 1809.

93 Jones, J., *Plain, Concise, Practical Remarks on the Treatment of Wounds and Fractures*, Robert Bell, Philadelphia, Pennsylvania, 1776.

94 Waters, N. B., *System of Surgery* (Extracted from The Works of Benjamin Bell) printed by T. Dobson, Philadelphia, 1791.

95 Cocke, W., *Inaugural Dissertation on Tetanus*, printed by R. Aitken, Philadelphia, 1798.

96 Bell, B., *System of Surgery*, London, 1750.

97 Dorsey, J. S., *Elements of Surgery*, published by Parker, E. and R., and Benjamin Warner, Philadelphia, 1818.

98 Dorsey, J. S., *Elements of Surgery*, published by Parker, E. and R., and Benjamin Warner, Philadelphia, 1818.

99 Bell, B., *System of Surgery*, London, 1750.

100 Packard, F. R., *The Practice of Medicine in the Northeast Colonies* (Quote of Ed Stafford, London, May 6, 1643), Journal American Medical Association, May 7, 1898.

101 Waters, N. B., *System of Surgery* (Extracted from the Works of Benjamin Bell) printed by T. Dobson, Philadelphia, 1791.

102 Bell, B., *Systems of Surgery*, London, 1750.

103 Black, R., *Inaugural Dissertation on Fractures*, printed by Ormrad and Conrad, Philadelphia, 1797.

104 Jones, J., Plain, *Concise, Practical Remarks on Treatment of Wounds and Fractures*, printed by R. Bell, Philadelphia, 1776.

105 Ibid.

106 Monro, J. K., Brit J. Surg 23, pp. 257-66, 1936.

107 Bell, B., *System of Surgery*, London, 1750.

108 Jones, J., *Plain, Concise, Practical Remarks on Treatment of Wounds and Fractures*, printed by R. Bell, Philadelphia, 1776.

109 Waters, N. B., *Systems of Surgery*, Printed by T. Dobson, Philadelphia, 1791.

110 Dorsey, S. J., *Elements of Surgery*, printed by Parker E. and R., and Benjamin Warner, Philadelphia, 1818.

111 Parkinson, J., *Huntarian Reminiscences*, printed by Sherwood, Gilbert and Piper, London, 1833.

112 Norris, G. W., *On The Occurence of Non-Unions After Fractures*, The American Journal of the Medical Sciences, January, 1842.

113 Parkinson, J., *Huntarian Reminiscences*, printed by Sherwood, Gilbert and Piper, London, 1833.

114 Dorsey, S. J., *Elements of Surgery*, printed by Parker, E. and R., and Benjamin Warner, Philadelphia, 1818.

115 Middleton, W. S., *Annals of Medical History* (New Series), 1 no. 5, pp. 362-82, P. Hoeber, New York, 1928.

116 Jones, J., *Plain Concise, Practical Remarks on Treatment of Wounds and Fractures*, printed by R. Bell, Philadelphia, 1776.

117 Wagensteen, Owen H.; Smith, J.; Wagensteen, S. D., *Some Highlights of the History of Amputations*. Bulletin of Historical Medicine, XLI, 1967.

118 Wagensteen, Owen H.; Smith, J.; Wagensteen, S. D., *Some Highlights of the History of Amputations*. Bulletin of Historical Medicine, XLI, 1967.

119 LeDran, H. F., *Treatise on Reflections Drawn from Practice on Gun-Shot Wounds*, printed by John Clarke, London, 1743.

120 Black, R., *Inaugural Dissertation on Fractures*, printed by Ormrad and Conrad, Philadelphia, 1797.

121 Donnison, J., *Midwives and Medical Men*, Schoken Books, New York, 1977.

122 Exton, B., *System of Midwifery*, printed by Wm. Owens, London, 1751.

123 W:_____S_____, M.D., *Aristotle's Compleat and Experyen'd Midwife*, Made English (4th, Ed.), London, 1721.

124 Bracken, H., M.D., The Midwives Companion or a Treatise of Midwifery, Printed by J. Clarke, London, 1737.

125 Exton, B., *System of Midwifery*, printed by Wm. Owens, London, 1751.

126 Donnison, J., *Midwives and Medical Men*, Schoken Books, New York, 1977.

127 Spencer, R. H., *The History of British Midwifery from 1650-1800*. John Bale & Sons and Danielsson, Ltd., London, 1927.

128 Spencer, R. H., *The History of British Midwifery from 1650-1800*. John Bale & Sons and Danielsson, Ltd., London, 1927.

129 *The Petition of the Unborn Babes and the Censors of the Royal College of London*, Anonymous, printed for M. Cooper, London, 1751.

130 Manning, C., *Remarks on the Employment of Females aa Practitioners of Midwifery*, Reprint of Lecture given in Boston, 1820.

131 Hamilton, A., *Outline of the Theory and Practice of Midwifery*, Reprinted by T. Dobson, Philadelphia, 1790.

132 Ibid.

133 Receipt Book Coates, E., (Paschall, Mrs. Jos.), handwritten, Philadelphia.

134 Ulrich, L., *The Diary of Martha Ballard*, Vintage Press, New York, 1991.

135 An Old German Midwives Record of Susanne Muller, Edited by Learned, M.D. and Breda, C. F.

136 Toner, J. M., *Contributions to the Annals of Medical Education in the U.S. before and during the War of Independence*, Government Printing Office, Washington, D.C., 1874.

137 Packard, F., *Early Methods of Medical Education in North America*, Journal American Medical Association, March 25, 1899.

138 Bard, S., *Compendium on the Theory and Practice of Midwifery*, printed by Collins and Co., New York, 1819.

139 Hamilton, A., *Outline of the Theory and Practice of Midwifery*, reprinted by Thomas Dobson, Philadelphia, 1790.

140 Blanton, W. B., *Medicine in Virginia in the 18th Century*, Garrett and Massie, Richmond, 1931.

141 Miller, J., *Caesarian Section in Virginia, Annals of Medical History* (New Series) 10:1938.

142 Blanton, W. B., *Medicine in Virginia in the 18th Century*, Garrett and Massie, Richmond, 1931.

143 Stookey, B., *A History of Colonial Medical Education*, Charles C. Thomas, Springfield, Illinois, 1962.

144 Elliott, J., *A Complete Collection of the Medical and Psychological Works* of John Fothergill, printed by J. Walker, London, 1781.

145 Hubard, J. T., *An Inaugural Dissertation on Puerperal Fever*, printed by John Ormrad, 41 Chestnut Street, Philadelphia, 1798.

146 Archer, J., *Every Man is his Own Doctor*, printed by P. Lillicrux, London, 1772.

147 Colbatch, J., Medicine Made Easy, Printed by J. Roberts, London (about 1750).

148 Wesley, J., *Primitive Physick*, printed by R. Hawes, London, 1772.

149 Jameson, H., *American Domestick Medicine*, 2nd Edition, Published by the Author, Baltimore, 1818.

150 Brugis, T., *The Marrow of Physicke*, T. Whittacker, London, 1648.

151 Moncrief, J., *The Poor Man's Physician or Receipts of the famous John Moncrief*, printed by George Stewart, Edinburgh, 1716.

152 Samson, W., *Rational Physic and Family Dispensatory*, printed for J. Fletcher and Company, London, 1765.

153 Aikin, J., *Memoirs of Medicine*, (quoted from a medical text by Andrew Bode), Printed by J. Johnson, London, 1780.

154 Brugis, T., *The Marrow of Physicke*, printed by Whittacker, London, 1648.

155 Ibid.

156 Ibid.

157 Dover, T., *The Ancient Physician's Legacy to his Country*, H. Kent, London, 1742.

158 The Philadelphia Gazette.

159 Darlington, Wm., Memorial to John Bartram and Humphrey Marshall. Printed by Lindsay Philadelphia, 1849.

160 Goodman, N., Benjamin Rush, Physician and Citizen, University of Pennsylvania Press, Philadelphia, 1934.

161 no author, *Maxims on the Preservation of Health and the Prevention of Disease*, Lee and Company, Patient and Family Medicine, Baltimore, circa 1813.

162 Seybolt, R. F., *New England Journal of Medicine*, V. 202, pp. 1067-8, 1930.

163 Miller, G., Ciba Symposium, *Medical Education in Colonial America*, January 1947, Summit, New Jersey.

164 Carson, J., *A History of the Medical Department of the University of Pennsylvania*, Lindsay and Blakiston, Philadelphia, 1869.

165 Earle, A. S., *Surgery in America*, Selected Writings, W. B. Saunders, Philadelphia & London, 1965.

166 Josselyn, J., Gent, Printed for G. Woddoes on the Green Dragon in St. Paul's Churchyard, 1695. (H. Felter, MD.., Bulletin of the Lloyd Library, Reprod. Series 8, 1927.)

167 Green, S., *Notes on a Copy of Dr. Wm. Douglass' Almanack*, Cambridge University Press, John Wilson & Son, 1884.

168 Ibid.

169 J. Med. Soc., N.J., V.57 #8, August 1960, pp. 491-6.

170 Story, J., From the Journal of Thomas Story, printed at New Castle on the Tyne, 1747, quoted by Carson, J., A History of the Medical Department of the University of Pennsylvania, Lindsay and Blakiston, Philadelphia, 1869.

171 Waring, J., *History of Medicine in South Carolina*, South Carolina Medical Association, 1964.

172 Beck, J., *Medicine in the American Colonies*, Horn and Wallace, Albuquerque, New Mexico, 1966.

173 Toner, J. M., *Continuation to Medical Progress and Medical Education Before and During the War of Independence*, Government Printing Office, Washington, DC., 1874.

174 Beck, J., *Medicine in the America Colonies*, Horn and Wallace, Albuquerque, New Mexico, 1966.

175 Thacher, J., *Military Journal during the American Revolutionary War*, Cotton & Barnard, Boston, 1827.

176 Steiner, W. R., James Thacher, *an Erudite Physician*, Bulletin of History of Medicine, Vol 1, #5, June 1933.

177 Packard, F.R., *The Practice of Medicine in the Northwest Colonies*, Journal of American Medical Association, May 7, 1898.

178 Bell, W., *Medical Students and their Examiners*, Trans. College of Physicians of Philadelphia, 4th sec. V 21, 1953-4.

179 Bell, W., *Bulletin Hist. Med.*, v. 31, 1957, p. 442-453.

180 Blanco, R. L., *Physician of the American Revolution*, Jonathan Pott, Garland STPM Press, New York & London, 1979.

181 Norwood, W. F., *Medicine in the Era of the American Revolution*, Int. Record of Medicine, V 171, #7, July 1958.

182 Middleton, W.S., Medical History Essays, privately printed, 1935.

183 Waters, N. B., *System of Surgery*, (Condensed from Benjamin Bell), printed by T. Dobson, Philadelphia, 1791.

184 Jones, J., *Plain and Concise Remarks in the Treatment of Wounds and Fractures*, printed by R. Bell in Philadelphia, 1776.

185 Davis, N. S., *Medical Education and Instruction in the United States*, S. C. Greggs Co., Chicago, 1851.

186 Parkinson, J., *Hunterian Reminiscences*, Sherwood, Gilbert & Piper, London, 1833.

187 Bridenbaugh, C., *The Itinerarium of Dr. Alexander Hamilton*, 1744, North Carolina Press, Chapel Hill, North Carolina, 1948.

188 Blake, J. B., *Diseases and Medical Practice in Colonel America*, Int. Record of Medicine, 171, 1958.

189 LeDran, H., *Treatise or Reflections Drawn From The Practice on Gun-Shot Wounds*, Translated from French and printed by John Clarke, London, 1743.

190 Billroth, T., *Historical Studies on the Nature and Treatment of Gunshot Wounds from the Fifteenth Century to the Present Time, Berlin, 1859. Translated by C. P. Rhoads*, Yale Journal of Biology and Medicine 4, pp. 119-142, 1931-2.

191 Waters, N. B., *Condensation of Surgery by Benjamin Bell*, printed by Dobson, Philadelphia, 1791.

192 Johnson, T., *The Collected Works of Ambroise Paré* (Translated from the Latin from the first English Edition, Printed by Milford, London 1634; Printed by Milford House, Pound Ridge, New York, 1968.

193 Billroth, T., *Historical Studies on the Nature and Treatment of Gunshot Wounds from the Fifteenth Century to the Present Time, Berlin, 1859. Translated by C. P. Rhoads*, Yale Journal of Biology and Medicine 4, pp. 119-142, 1931-2.

194 Wangensteen, O. H., *Some Highlights in the History of Amputations*, Bulletin of History of Medicine V, XLI, March/April 1967.

195 Waters, N. B., *Condensation of Surgery by Benjamin Bell*, printed by Dobson, Philadelphia, 1791.

196 Jones, J., Plain, *Concise Remarks of Wounds and Fractures* (2nd Edition), printed by Dobson, Philadelphia, 1776

197 Ibid.

198 Earle, A., *Surgery in America*, W. B. Saunders, Philadelphia and London, 1965.

199 Pringle, J., *Observations of the Diseases of the Army*, 2nd Edition, Printed by E. Earle, Philadelphia, 1816.

200 Monro, D., *An Account of the Diseases Most Frequent in British Military Hospitals in Germany*, Printed by A. Mullar and D. Wilson, London, 1764.

201 Van Swieten, G., (Translated by John Ranley Surgeon General to the British Army), Printed by R. Bell, Philadelphia, 1776.

202 Rush, B., *Preserving the Health of Soldiers*, Printed by J. Dunlop, Lancaster, Pennsylvania, 1778.

203 *Collection of handwritten Letters between G. Washington and B. Rush*, College of Physicians, Philadelphia.

204 Middleton, W., Annals of Medical History, 3rd Series, VIII, No. 5, 1941, p 461.

205 Cash, P., *Medical Men at the Siege of Boston*, American Philosophical Society, Boston, 1973.

206 Lewis, F., *Medicine in the Continental Army of the Revolutionary War*, Senior Thesis for Department of History, Princeton University, New Jersey, 1956.

207 Carlson, E., Bulletin New York Academy of Medicine, V 55, No.7, July/Aug, 1979.

208 Hamilton, R., *Duties of a Regimental Surgeon*, Vol I & II, printed by George Woodfall, London, 1787.

209 Ibid.

210 Bayne-Jones, S., *The Evolution of Preventive Medicine in the U.S. Army* 1607-1939, Office of the Surgeon General, Washington, DC, 1968.

211 Cantlie, N., *History of Medicine*, Department of the British Army, Longmans, Green, London.

212 Ibid.

213 Collection of Letters of G. Washington and B. Rush, College of Physicians of Philadelphia.

214 Woods, A., Delaware Medical Journal, V44, No.3, p.59, March 1972.

215 Ibid.

216 *Journal of the Continental Congress*, 1774-83.

217 Duncan, L. D., *Medical Memoirs in the America Revolution* 1775-83, A. Kelley, New York, 1970.

218 Davis, D., *Medicine in the Canadian Campaign of the Revolutionary War*, Bulletin of History of Medicine, V44, p. 461, 1970.

219 Senter, I., *The Journal of Isaac Senter*, Historical Society of Pennsylvania, 1846.

220 Thacher, J., *Military Journal During the Revolutionary War from 1775-1783*, Cotton and Bernard, Boston, 1827.

221 Senter, I., *The Journal of Isaac Senter*, Historical Society of Pennsylvania, Philadelphia,1846.

222 Ibid.

223 Davis, D., *Medicine in the Canadian Campaign of the Revolutionary War*, Journal of Dr. John Fist Merrick, Bulletin of History of Medicine, V44, pp. 241-76, 1970.

224 Duncan, L., *Medical Men in the American Revolution*, Augustus M. Kelley, New York, 1970.

225 Ibid.

226 Ibid.

227 Wooden, A., Delaware Medical Journal, V 44, No. 3, pp. 39-65, March 1972.

228 Thacher, J., *American Medical Biography*, printed by Richardson and Lord, and Cotton's and Bernard, Boston, 1828.

229 Duncan, L., Medical *Men in the American Revolution 1775-1783*, A. Kelley, New York, 1970.

230 Thacher, J., *Military Journal During the Revolutionary War from 1775-1783*, Cotton, Bernard, Boston, 1827.

231 Jones, J., *Plain, Concise, Practical Treatment of Wounds and Fractures* (2nd Edition), printed by Dobson, Philadelphia, 1776.

232 Thacher, J., *Military Journal During the Revolutionary War from 1775-1783*, Cotton, Bernard, Boston, 1827.

233 Blanco, R., *Physician of the American Revolution*, Jonathon Potts, Garland STPM Press, New York & London, 1979.

234 Reid, M., *The Mohawk Valley*, It's Legends and It's History, New York and London, 1901.

235 LeDran, H., *Treatise or Reflection Drawn From The Practice of Gun-Shot Wounds*, Translated from French and printed by John Clarke, London, 1743.

236 Duncan, L, *Medical Men in the American Revolution 1775-1783*, A. Kelley, New York, 1970.

237 Duncan, L, *Medical Men in the American Revolution 1775-1783*, A. Kelley, New York, 1970.

238 Ibid.

239 Gibson, J., Annals of Medical History, (New Series 10), pp. 382-9, 1938.

240 Waters, N. B., *Condensation of Surgery by Benjamin Bell*, printed by Dobson, Philadelphia, 1791.

241 Northcote, W., *The Diseases Incident to the Armies with the Method of Cure by Baron Von Swieten*, included in Brief Directions to be Observed by Sea Surgeons in Engagements, Printed by R. Bell, Philadelphia, 1776.

242 Ibid.

243 Ibid.

244 Northcote, W., Extracts for the Marine Practice of Physics and Surgery for the Use of Military and Naval Surgeons in America, R. Bell, Philadelphia, 1776.

245 Blanco, R. H., *Medicine in the Continental Army*, Bulletin of New York Academy of Medicine, V 57, pp. 677-704, 1981.

246 Owen, W., *Medical Department of the U. S. Army*, Paul Hoeber, New York, 1920.

247 Blanco, R., *Medicine in the Continental Army*, 1775-1781, Bulletin of New York Academy Medicine, V 57, 1981.

248 Cowen, D., *Medicine in Revolutionary New Jersey*, New Jersey Historical Commission, 1975.

249 Public Record Office, W.O.1/683 (313-653); W.O.4/725 (51-61), London.

250 Cowen, D., *Medicine in Revolutionary New Jersey*, New Jersey Historical Commission, 1975.

251 Duncan, L., *Medical Men in the American Revolution*, Augustus Kelley, New York, 1970.

252 Norcross, W., *The Enigma of Benjamin Church*, Medical Arts & Sciences, 2nd Quart., 1956.

253 Norcross, W., *The Enigma of Benjamin Church*, Medical Arts & Sciences, 2nd Quart., 1956.

254 Ibid.

255 Miller, R. G., *Medical Education in Colonial America*, Ciba Symposium, Summit, New Jersey, January 1947.

256 Heiges, G., *Letters Relating to Colonial Military Hospital in Lancaster County*, Lancaster County Historical Society, V-LIII, No. 4, 1948.

257 Ibid.

258 Ibid.

259 Heiges, G., *Letters Relating to Colonial Military Hospital in Lancaster County*, Lancaster County Historical Society, V-LII, No. 4, 1948.

260 Owen, W., *Medical Department of the U. S. Army*, Paul Hoeber, New York, 1920.

261 Tilton, J., *Oeconomical Observations on Military Hospitals and the Prevention and Cure of Diseases Incident to the Army*, printed by Wilson, Wilmington, Delaware, 1813.

262 Packard, F. R., *The Care of the Sick and Wounded in the Revolution* (An address before the Judson Daland Society delivered January 8, 1899), reprinted from North Carolina Medical Journal, Charlotte, North Carolina.

263 Packard, F. R., *The Care of the Sick and Wounded in the Revolution* (An address before the Judson Daland Society delivered January 8, 1899), reprinted from North Carolina Medical Journal, Charlotte, North Carolina.

264 Packard, F. R., *The Care of the Sick and Wounded in the Revolution* (An address before the Judson Daland Society delivered January 8, 1899), reprinted from North Carolina Medical Journal, Charlotte, North Carolina.

265 Packard, F. R., *The Care of the Sick and Wounded in the Revolution* (An address before the Judson Daland Society delivered January 8, 1899), reprinted from North Carolina Medical Journal, Charlotte, North Carolina.

266 Beck, J., *Medicine in the American Colonies*, Horn & Lovelace, Albuquerque, New Mexico, 1966.

267 Owen, W., *Medical Department of the U. S. Army*, Paul Hoeber, New York, 1920.

268 Owen, W., *Medical Department of the U. S. Army*, Paul Hoeber, New York, 1920.

269 Journal of Continental Congress 1774-83.

270 Pringle, J., *Observations of the Diseases of Armies*. 1st American Edition, Edward Earle, Philadelphia, 1810.

271 Aikin, J., Thoughts on Hospitals, printed by J. Johnson, London, 1771.

272 Von Swieten, G., *Diseases Incident to Armies with the Method of Cure*.

273 Jones, J., *Plain Concise, Practical Remarks on Treatment of Wounds*, printed by R. Bell, 1776, Philadelphia.

274 Butterfield, L. H., *Letters of Benjamin Rush to the Officers in the Army of the United American States: Directions for Preserving the Health of Soldiers*, American Philosophical Society, Princeton University Press, 1951.

275 Butterfield, L. H., *Letters of Benjamin Rush to the Officers in the Army of the United American States: Directions for Preserving the Health of Soldiers*, American Philosophical Society, Princeton University Press, 1951.

276 Ibid.

277 Ibid.

278 Tilton, J., *Oeconomical Observations on Military Hospitals and the Prevention and Cure of Diseases Incident to the Army*, printed by Wilson, Wilmington, Delaware, 1813.

279 Cantile, N., *History of the British Army Medical Department*, Vol 1, Churchill, Livingtone, London, 1974.

280 Duncan, L., *Medical Men in the American Revolution*, Augustus Kelley, New York, 1970.

281 Gordon, M., *Naval and Maritime Medicine During the American Revolution*, Ventnor Publishers, Ventnor, New Jersey, 1978.

282 Cantile, N., *History of the British Army Medical Department*, Vol 1, Churchill, Livingtone, London, 1974.

283 Ibid.

284 Peckham, H., *The Toll of Independence*, University of Chicago Press, Chicago, 1974.

285 Duncan, L.C., *Medical Men in the American Revolution*, Augustus Kelley, New York, 1970.

286 *Personal Mimeograph*, Baltimore, 1959.

287 Aikin, J., *Thoughts on Hospitals*, Printed by J. Johnson, London, 1771.

288 Ibid.

289 Ibid.

290 Jones, J., *Plain, Concise, Practical Remarks on Treatment of Wounds and Fractures*, Printed by Robert Bell, Philadelphia, 1776.

291 Aikin, J., *Thoughts on Hospitals*, Printed by J. Johnson, London, 1771.

292 Jones, J., Plain, *Concise, Practical Remarks on Treatment of Wounds and Fractures*, Printed by Robert Bell, Philadelphia, 1776.

293 Aikin, J., *Thoughts on Hospitals*, Printed by J. Johnson, London, 1771.

294 Ibid.

295 Tilton, J., *Oeconomical Observations on Military Hospitals*, Printed by Wilson, Wilmington, Delaware, 1813.

296 Pringle, J., *Observations in the Diseases of the Army*, 1752. Republished by Earle, Philadelphia, 1810.

297 Shryock, R., *Empiricum vs. Rationalism in America*, Reprinted from the Proceedings of American Medical Antiquarian Society, Worcester, Mass., April 1969.

298 Bridenbaugh, C., *Dr. Thomas Bond's Essays on the Utility of Clinical Lectures*, Journal of History of Medicine and Applied Sciences, V2, 1947.

299 Duer, W. A., *Reminiscences of an Old New Yorker*, W. L. Andrews, New York, NY, 1967. Reprinted from American Mail, No.5, July 3, 1847.

300 Butterfield, L. H., Benjamin Rush's *Reminiscences of Boswell and Johnson 1765*. Princeton University Press, 1951.

301 Hindle, B., *The Pursuit of Science in America*. University of North Carolina Press, Chapel Hill, 1956.

302 Earle, A., *Surgery in America*; Selected Writings. W. B. Saunders, Philadelphia/ London, 1965.

303 Lettson, J., *Works of John Fothergill*, M.D. Vol 1, Printed by Chas. Dilley, London, 1783.

304 Ibid.

305 Thacher, J., *American Medical Biography, 1st Edition*. Richardson and Lord, Boston, 1828.

306 Lining, J., *Philosophical Transaction XLII*. T. Woodward Company, London, 1744.

307 Heberden, W., *Observations on the Increase and Decrease of Disease.* L. Hanford, London, 1801.

308 Hardie, J., *Account of the Malignant Fever in the City of New York.* Printed by Hurtin and McFarland, New York, 1799.

309 Webster, N., *Collection of Papers on Bilious Fever.* Hopkins & Webb, New York, 1796.

310 Hunter, J., *Diseases of the Army in Jamaica*, T. Payne 3rd ed., London, 1808.

311 Parkinson, J., *Hunterian Reminiscences.* Sherwood, Albert, Piper, London, 1833.

312 Pringle, J., A Discourse on the Different Kind of Air: address delivered to Royal Academy on November 30, 1773. Printed by Royal Academy, London, 1774.

313 Ibid.

314 *Minutes of the Common Council of the City* of New York 1, 208, 1689.

315 Heaton, C., *Bulletin History of Medicine*, V17, pp. 217-37, 1945.

316 Ibid.

317 Cogressi, C., *New Theory of Contagious Diseases Among Oxen.* Seizone Lombarda Della Docieta, Italiano di Microbiologica, Rome, 1953.

318 Andrey, N., *An Account of Breeding of Worms in Human Bodies.* H. Rhodes, London, 1701.

319 Marten, B., *A New Theory of Consumption.* Knaplock, London, 1722.

320 Nuttal, G., *Parasitology*, V18, pp. 398-407, 1921.

321 Bean, W., *Jefferson's Influence on Medical Education.* Virginia Medical Monthly, V87, December, 1960.

322 Jefferson, T., *The Writings of Thomas Jefferson.* Thomas Jefferson Memorial Association XVI, Washington, D.C., 1905.

323 Purchas, S., *Purchas*, His Pilgrims. Printed by W. S. Henry, 1619.

324 Rush, B., *Apprentices to Dr. Rush.* Manuscript, College of Physicians, Philadelphia, 1812.

325 Ibid.

326 Home, E., *Treatice on the Blood, Inflammation by John Hunter*. Printed by T. Bradford, Philadelphia, 1796.

327 Pringle, J., *Observations on the Diseases of the Army*. Published by E. Earle, Philadelphia, 1810.

328 Jones, J., *Plain Concise Remarks on Treatment of Wounds & Fractures*. Robert Bell, Philadelphia, 1776.

329 Tilton, J., *Oeconomical Observations on Military Hospitals and the Prevention and Cure of Disease*. Wilson, Wilmington, Delaware, 1813.

330 Waters, N., *System of Surgery*. Dobson, Philadelphia, 1791.

331 Pringle, J., *First American Edition with notes by Benjamin Rush*. Published by Edward Earle, Philadelphia, 1810.

332 Alexander, W., *Experimental Essays*. Printed for E.& C. Dilley, London, 1768.

333 Reese, D., *Humbugs of New York*, J. S. Taylor, Boston, 1838.

334 Perkins, B., *The Influence of Metallic Tractors on the Human Body*, printed gby J. Johnson, London, 1799.

335 Thacher, J., *American Medical Biography*, Vol. I. First Edition, Boston, 1828; DaCapo Press, New York, 1967.

336 Billroth, T., *Treatment of Gunshot Wounds from the Fifteenth Century to the Present*. Translated by C. P. Rhoad, Yale Journal of Biology and Medicine, 4, pp. 119-142, 1931-2.

337 Ibid.

338 Ibid.

339 Gooch, B., *The Chirurgical Works of Benjamin Gooch*, Surgeon V-III. Printed by J. Johnson, London, 1792.

340 Home, E., *A Treatise on the Blood, Inflammation and Gunshot Wounds*. Printed by Thomas Bradford, Philadelphia, 1796.

341 Parkinson, J., *Hunterian Reminiscences*. Being the Substance of a Course of Lectures by John Hunter. Sherwood, Gilbert, Piper, London, 1833.

342 Ibid.

343 Norris, G., *American Journal of the Medical Sciences*, January, 1842.

344 LeDran, H., *Treatise or Reflections Drawn from Practice on Gun-Shot Wounds.* Printed by J. Clarke, London, 1743.

345 Butler, J., *Lectures in Surgery by Philip S. Physick & John Dorsey.* Hand Written Copybook of J. Butler. College of Physicians, Philadelphia, 1809.

346 Earle, A., *Surgery in America; Selected Writings.* W. B. Saunders, Philadelphia/ London, 1965.

INDEX